Voices of the
Soft-bellied
Warrior

Also by Mary Saracino

Finding Grace
No Matter What

Voices of the Soft-bellied Warrior

A Memoir

Mary Saracino

Spinsters Ink Books
Denver, Colorado
USA

First edition published October 2001
10-9-8-7-6-5-4-3-2-1

Spinsters Ink Books
P. O. Box 22005
Denver, CO 80222
USA

Edited by Joan M. Drury
Copy edit by Paulette Whitcomb
Cover sculpture by Mary Saracino
Cover design by Attention Media Group
Cover photo by Leav Bolender
Interior design by Gilsvik Book Production
Publicity by Claire Kirch Publicity Services

Production:
Katherine Hovis
Nina Miranda
Sharon Silvas

Library of Congress Cataloging-in-Publication Data

Saracino, Mary, 1954—
    Voices of the soft-bellied warrior: a memoir/Mary Saracino—1st ed.
    p. cm.
    ISBN 1-883523-41-9
    1. Saracino, Mary, 1954— 2. Novelists, American—20th century—Biography.
3. Incest victims—United States—Biography. 4. Voice disorders—Patients—
Biography. 5. Authorship—Psychological aspects. I. Title.

PS3569.A65 Z47 2001
813'.54—dc21
[B]

Acknowledgments

This memoir was born of great strife and deep healing. Through four years of not knowing what was happening to my voice, I encountered numerous compassionate people who helped lighten my journey. To each of them I owe a debt of gratitude. I especially wish to thank Teresa Saracino, Peg Saracino Sutherland, and Cheryl Hagen for their unconditional love and generosity of spirit.

I am deeply grateful to my life partner Jane Butz and two gifted healers, Laura Lucas-Silvis and Patricia Schuckert, for witnessing and blessing my life in deep and lasting ways. Each of these women continually encouraged me to mend my broken places, break the silence, and speak my truth.

I am indebted to Joan Drury for helping this book become a reality. She is truly its midwife. As the former owner of Spinsters Ink, Joan accepted the original manuscript and, after selling the press, continued to champion its pages to Spinsters' new owners, Sharon Silvas and Kathy Hovis. Blessedly, Sharon and Kathy listened and agreed. Without Joan's tireless belief in the goodness and value of *Voices of the Soft-bellied Warrior* the book might not have been published. As the book's editor, I also wish to thank her for her careful eye, open heart, and unfailing belief in the importance of women's stories. Molto grazie, Joan.

I wish to thank Sharon and Kathy at Spinsters Ink for allowing my book to be their first. Many thanks, as well, to the savvy team of talented and committed people who ushered the manuscript through all of its pre and post publication stages—Tracy Gilsvik, Grant Dunmire, Paulette Whitcomb, Claire Kirch, and Nina Miranda.

And always, loving gratitude to my grandmothers—Fiora Vergamini and Immacolata Saracino. Tanti baci, nonne. E millie grazie per tutto.

This book is for Jane Butz and Laura Lucas-Silvis

"When we accept our body and our feelings, we treat them in an affectionate, nonviolent way . . . we do not turn ourselves into a battlefield with the good side fighting the bad. When we can see the non-duality of the rose and the garbage, the roots of affliction and the awakened mind, we are no longer afraid."

—Reprinted from *Transformation and Healing:*
Sutra on the Four Establishments of Mindfulness
(1990) by Thich Nhat Hanh with permission of
Parallax Press, Berkeley, California

Author's Note

This memoir is an amalgam of my personal experiences, dreams, and interactions with others. As such, it is told from my singular point-of-view. Although I have changed many (but not all) of the names, I have endeavored to write factually of my experience as I perceived it. Others may recall shared events differently; that is the nature of human memory and individual perspective. My intention was to write my truth as I knew it to be.

$\mathcal{S}$hortly before my first novel, *No Matter What*, was published in September 1993, I began to have difficulty speaking. At first, I noticed a slight impairment. A tight vowel sound here, a fuzzy consonant there. Gradually, over a period of six months, my voice worsened, making it difficult for me to talk and to function in the world. I had no idea what was causing this impediment. I grew increasingly frustrated that it should arise at this most important and exciting juncture in my life. I had a book to promote. I needed to rely on my voice more than ever before.

Eventually, all my speech became labored. By March 1994, my voice had surrendered to this mystery ailment. My throat became a vise of tight muscles as I fought to release my words. My vocal cords would not cooperate. I could no longer talk or read out loud without immense struggle. I stopped doing public readings of *No Matter What*.

"Do you have a cold?" people would ask me. On the phone, in person, people I knew, perfect strangers. I'd recoil in shame. My voice had exposed me. I couldn't hide from my problem.

What exactly was the problem? I knew I had trouble speaking. I could plainly hear that. But why?

I had no clue.

While I was elated and reeling from the success of realizing my lifelong dream of being an author, I was also in a great deal of emotional pain. *No Matter What* is semi-autobiographical, based in part on a traumatic childhood experience. The writing of it, I reasoned, had touched deep unhealed wounds, holding my voice hostage. How ironic that at a time I was beginning to come into the full power of my writer's voice and break the silence of my childhood abuse, I should lose my speaking voice.

In 1993 when my speech problems were minor compared to what they would eventually become, I sought out a voice instructor. With my publication date looming and the prospect of public readings before me, I felt compelled to find a solution. Fast.

I told my voice teacher about my speaking problem. We practiced making sounds together. She taught me how to improve my breathing and focus my energy on my solar plexus. She helped ease my rising performance anxiety. I learned how to meditate. I practiced reading my work out loud and breathing. That got me through the publication party and my first public reading.

After that, I did more readings at more bookstores. These offered me more chances to meditate, breathe, read. Sometimes my voice would crack; sometimes the words would flow with less friction than before, but always there was static in my head and in my heart. I didn't sound good enough. Friends would comfort, "It's not as bad as you think." I didn't believe them. I could hear the vowel breaks, the consonants that refused to cooperate. I could feel the audience's eyes on me, and it felt as if I was falling deeper and deeper into an abyss of voicelessness.

The combination of impaired speech and spiraling shame was toxic. I decided to return to psychotherapy in order to confront the issues that I believed were strangling my voice. Certain that unhealed emotional wounds had arisen during the writing of my novel, I had no doubt that on a subconscious level I was trying to silence myself.

My psychotherapist recommended a speech therapist. The speech therapist decided my problem was tongue placement. For six months, I practiced the exercises he gave me. I did vowel slides and stretched my lips with small rubber tubing. I repeated tongue twister sentences and strings of phrases meant to re-train my tongue to improve airflow and create proper voicing. In the end, the routine eased the terrible muscle tension in my neck, but the quality of my voice did not change substantially. I sounded good in the speech therapist's office when I only had to speak in a controlled environment, but out in the real world, I clenched.

I quit speech therapy and continued psychotherapy. I followed my natural inclination to explore alternative forms of healing. I did bodywork. I continued to meditate. I tried acupuncture and a multitude of herbal remedies trying to find the "cure" for my worsening voice. I felt healthier and more balanced than ever before in my life, but I still couldn't talk.

I dove into psychotherapy, fully committed to uncovering the body-mind connection that was imprisoning my voice. I healed a lot of unfinished business. The novel *had* stirred up old ghosts; I hadn't dreamed that part.

I struggled through therapy, unable to vocalize most of my

feelings. Traditional talk approaches were impossible. My therapist and I found a way to conquer this obstacle. I drew pictures, painted paintings, sculpted clay figures, wrote poems and letters to access my feelings, communicate my experience. In doing so, I unearthed the subconscious mother lode of my inner life.

My journey to uncover what was awry with my speaking voice unexpectedly took a deeper turn. The healing I was seeking was more than physiological. There was a hidden pilgrimage inside the obvious one. Losing my speaking voice had messy repercussions. My insistent yearning for ease in speech mirrored a more organic need to heal the wounds of my childhood and be heard—as a writer and artist and as a woman in recovery from childhood abuse.

Even as I faced my personal demons, my speaking voice refused to budge.

By the fall of 1996, I was physically, emotionally, and spiritually distraught. I felt exhausted, frustrated, angry, and deeply grieved that all my earnest attempts to uncover the root of my voice problem had come to no avail. I was seriously depressed. Crying without reason. Afraid of the world. I cringed at the smallest, briefest encounters with others because I would be expected to talk.

I found myself unable and unwilling to connect with people —except through the written word. I withdrew. My relationship suffered. My friendships suffered. My self-esteem suffered. I discontinued public readings, so the promotion of my novel suffered, as well. By some miraculous act of grace, my freelance-writing clients didn't desert me, so I could still support myself.

Off and on through the process I tried St. John's Wort, Bach Flower remedies, Chinese herbal-pill anxiety remedies. Everything helped relieve the anxiety and depression for a few weeks, but nothing proved to have lasting power. I finally met with a Western medical doctor and started taking the anti-depressant Paxil. It helped. A lot. Emotionally restored, I was able to engage in my life with more ease and confidence. My inner voice felt strong and vibrant, loud and clear. However, my speaking voice still wasn't back to its original state.

Seven months later, I went to my family doctor in desperation. She referred me to an ear, nose and throat (ENT) specialist to determine if I had polyps on my vocal cords, or worse—a malignant tumor.

The ENT examined my vocal cords. No polyps. No tumor. She suspected something she called *spasmodic dysphonia*—a rare voice disorder in which the basal ganglia, deep in the brain, miscue and inappropriately send neurotransmitters to stimulate the vocal cord muscles to contract. The result is strangled speech. There's no cure, she told me, but there was a treatment.

Finally. I had the answer I had been waiting years to hear. I had a *real* medical condition. A voice disorder. It wasn't fatal or curable, but there was a physical reason I couldn't talk. And a way to treat this rare anomaly.

This memoir is about my journey back home to my voice. During the four years of not knowing what was happening to my speech, I kept a journal of my experiences, thoughts, feelings, and dreams. I also painted and sculpted. Although traditional Western medical doctors might see spasmodic dysphonia as purely physical in nature, I experienced it differently.

Something *is* awry in the basal ganglia of my brain. However, I believe that my mind, spirit, and body all played a part in bringing me to this point.

Science tells us that emotions are biochemical reactions, and if one examines the body merely as a physical entity, separate and apart from the soul, I agree. Every physical process can be extrapolated into its cellular functions. Memory, feelings, ideas—indeed consciousness itself—are biochemical. Still, the body possesses a consciousness separate and distinct from (yet connected to) its mental and emotional counterparts.

Like my mind, my body has a memory, a history. Whatever trauma or jubilation it has experienced has manifested itself, in one way or another, in the emotional/physical/spiritual ecosystem known as me.

Writing *No Matter What* turned the knob, freeing me to enter another dimension of my psyche. It also unleashed long-held emotional wounds that my body had stored and protected for over thirty years. Did this trigger the spasmodic dysphonia? I believe so. For whatever reason, the basal ganglia are the weakest link in my body-mind-spirit chain. Is it a coincidence that I was physically silenced as I was shattering emotional lies? I don't think so.

From an early age, I was trained to be a secret keeper, at grave cost to my own well-being. At some point, my system broke down or rebelled or blew a circuit. However one wishes to describe it, the fact remains that my particular system-overload resulted in spasmodic dysphonia. Some other person's might have manifested itself as arthritis or cancer or multiple sclerosis.

My road to wellness began when I grew able to see that the disparate and disheveled tiles of my life fit into one intricately remarkable mosaic. By excavating the discarded shards of my self, I learned to restore the delicate balance of my life. I still have a voice disorder, but I am richer for it, in myriad intangible ways. I finally understand that while I can't *fix* my voice, I can open my heart to my life's contradictions and try, every day, to embrace the paradoxes I find there.

This is one woman's story of discovery and epiphany.

This is my story. The autobiography of my voice.

Through four years of strangled speech, I excavated the vein of my subconscious searching for the sound of my fury. I painted images with watercolors and oil pastels. I sculpted warriors out of clay. These soft-bellied archetypal female figures, with mouths open wide, dared to shout my truths. When my physical voice was impaired, my hands learned to articulate the language of healing.

Artwork and dreams brought me out of silence. Soft-bellied warriors carried me home.

1994

Chapter 1

There is a psychic cord tethering me to my mother. It is thick and heavy. It wraps its prickly fingers around the soft skin of my throat. When I was a child, I made a tacit agreement with my mother to keep my family's secrets. Protect her at all costs. I have paid a high price for this silencing.

My voice is raw. My emotions stretched to a thin slit of air, a violin string taut against the bones in my neck, screeching its painful aria. My voice is on fire. It flares with ferocious rage. It bites and singes, eating away the flesh of my will to live.

I am afraid to meet the world. Fearful of ordinary, everyday encounters at the grocery store, at the gas station, friendly greetings as I walk around Lake Harriet. I am afraid to open my mouth and speak because each time I do not know what will come forth. Every hello is fragmented, frayed, fraught with tension and strangled consonants, mangled vowels.

I am afraid of my writing. What has chosen me feeds the desperate flames of my struggle to voice my truth. I write of old wounds, unhealed grief, stories that are stored in my bones, my blood, the very fiber of my cell walls. I excavate the mother lode of memory and polish the rough stones into imperfect facets, reflecting the pain and the joys of my life. Will what I write emerge in a clear sweet voice, fluid and honest? Or will the sentences and paragraphs grate against the grasping voice of stagnant secrets? This emotional wound has caused impairment. My physical voice is strained. I can no longer trust my vocal cords. And so, too, I can no longer trust the vocal folds of my inner, writer's voice to bellow this insistent necessity: break the silences.

I feel the full power of my mother's hand around my throat, but now the fingers have become mine, clutching, clenching, and shoving the truth into my belly.

I try to open to this challenge, loosen the clenched fingers of muscle that throttle my speech asking me to wake up, shake myself free from this vise of silence. I want to disown my ugly voice. Pretend it is not mine. I want to blame my mother, say it is her fault, her needs that this airless stranglehold serves. But mine are served, too. My need to be protected. My need to silence the big body emotions that course through my cells. They wait to shout their truth. Will I die if I let myself unleash the backlog?

Mama came first. Always and forever. Don't rock the boat. Be good. Mama loves you more than anyone. Of course there were conditions. *I will love you if you do not remind me of my pain. I will love you if you do what I tell you to do. I will love you if you keep*

4

your mouth shut. Don't tell me about your grief, about your isolation, your abandonment. Don't say the things that Mama cannot bear to hear.

Why does she get to be crazy full of pain, but I don't?

Mama pulls the cord tighter. I cannot speak. Each time I try, I am silenced by her tearful looks, her wounded heart, my own acquiescence. How could I hurt her?

I want to loosen the cord. Remove it. Feel the wind sting the raw, red burns on my throat. I no longer accept this unspoken agreement. I have outgrown its purpose. I reach for the long-bladed knife. I cut the rope, lick my sores clean. Wait for the scar tissue to bind my old skin to my new.

I am tired. I feel as if I am unable to hold my head up. I am weary.

I want to write again. I am drained and empty, spiritually anemic from not writing. I have been punishing myself for writing my novel, *No Matter What.* It causes trouble in my family's emotional life. My parents, my siblings, my aunts and uncles, my stepfather have to relive the past, nurse their grief. It is a nuisance. I wrote about my life as a young girl lost in a family falling apart. I broke the silence of my mother's affair with a parish priest. I told the truth of how I was her confidante, bearing too much for my young girl's shoulders. Though the nitty-gritty details of *No Matter What* are primarily fictionalized, the emotional reality of my life as my mother's daughter surfaces as the truest autobiographical component of the novel.

I feel exposed and very bad, bad, bad. I am trying to free myself from the tyranny of my own self-negation. Self-censorship. Silencing. *Be good at all costs.* That has always been my motto. The costs are high when I write, but the costs to myself are higher if I do not. I am bound in a terrible knot of frustration. If I betray myself by setting down my writing pen, others breathe easier. But

5

I become miserable. I am literally unable to speak. My physical voice is traumatized. What do I have to lose? If I write, I can free my voice, both my physical ability to speak and be heard, and the metaphorical voice of my craft. If I don't write I lose precious time. I commit spiritual suicide. I must try to find a way. For my own sanity. For my own personal necessity.

I gave my therapist, Anne, a copy of *No Matter What.* It was hard to ask her to read my book and tell her what it was about. I felt exposed—afraid she would find my pain disgusting, my book as something better left unwritten. Why did I write it? Why was I compelled to tell? Get the truth out? And why did I leave out the incest? Am I punishing myself for writing it? Is that what this strangled speech is about? Is my voice clenching because I am trying to stop myself from reading out loud the truth of my own life?

This grieving aches. The memories won't let me be. Do they define me? Limit me? Or just contribute to who and what I am? I run from the pain and when I stop running, it is still there. And the book is still there. My book. My voice. My pain. Waiting to be honored by me. Can I love the part of me that wrote the book? If I am a messenger, what am I trying to tell myself? And why is it so hard to listen? My heart hurts from the noise of it all. I want to scream and scream and scream. Then it will come out, all the horrible, wretched pain, the thick dark blood of it all. And if I scream and scream and scream, what will happen? Will my mother collapse into a coma? Will she feel the terrible weight of her own choices? If I drop the burden, if I give it back, will she take it up, hold it tight and know it as her own? If she doesn't, do I have to pick it up again? Do I have to carry the secrets for my family?

I am the bad girl. I broke my promise. I told the world and now they all know. Does that make *me* the monster? I am the evil one, the one who can't keep her mouth shut. The one whose head and heart swell with the need to tell. Tell on them. Heal myself.

Wake up.

I was groomed to be a good girl. The ground rules were simple: never express the hard feelings, the rage, the anger, the deep grieving, the crabby, terrible side. I stuff, hide, pretend those parts do not exist. But they are knocking on my door now, telling me they want in. They want to make me complete and complex and fully human. They have been in exile too long. They want to come home. *That's* why I wrote *No Matter What.* I feel fractured, incomplete, wanting the murky shadow side to reintegrate but fearing it. How will it change my identity to not always be the good, kind, sweet girl with a heart of selfless gold? Are the hard feelings the real gold? Am I bankrupt?

I dreamt I was making art using black beans, brown rice, and beets—natural organic products and dyes—as my materials. I was creating a mosaic about incest and its emotional impact on children and on the adults abused children grow to be. I was outside at Lake of the Isles, making my art in a public place at a picnic table by the shore. People joined me, and I moved my art materials to make space for them. The people started eating some of the foodstuffs I had brought to use in my art. "Pass me the brown rice," they said. "I want more black beans." "I want beets." I hesitated, wanting to hoard my materials. I needed the beets to make a dark purple-red dye for blood and pain and grief. But I passed the food to the people, and they ate. A man asked me about my art. I told him I was making a mosaic about incest and its impact on my life. I felt strong and confident, empowered by the image I was creating. In the dream, my voice was clear and strong. I was not afraid. I felt at ease and confident and good, sharing my art in public.

It is raining. The drizzle never stops. It is heavy, this early autumn grieving. It reminds me of *that* autumn—September 1967—when my mother took my sisters and me and left my father and my four brothers. We buried our sadness that day, and all the days after. Stiff lips and stiff legs. Hurting hearts trying so hard to hold it all in. I ached to disappear. Somehow I thought the pain would go away when we left. All the heartache from living in that house on Bayard Street. All the confusion of leading parallel lives—one with my sisters and brothers, my father and mother, the other with my mother and my sisters and the man my mother loved. The pain of the incest. The pain of growing up in terror. I thought our leaving would cleanse me. I didn't count on the strength of the ties that connected me to my brothers and to my father. Over a thousand miles of hills and highways, rivers and lakes separated me from my hometown, my blood ties. Over a thousand strands of genetic memory, cultural identity, cellular longings for something that could no longer be.

I have been journaling as part of what Julia Cameron called "morning pages" in her book *The Artist's Way*. In a way, it is cleansing. Like mind-dumping, I liberate the creative force from its censor, that nasty foul-breathed imposter who tells me I can't continue because, because, because. A thousand reasons. Fear keeps me immobilized. I want to break through. Julia Cameron wrote about the artist being one's inner child, that part of one's self still connected to emotions and magic, wonder and playfulness—even one's ugliest wounds. I need all of it. I can't run anymore.

Now, in my fortieth year, the challenge is to continue to heal the chronic wounds of my childhood, the sexual abuse, the emotional abandonment, my mother's affair, the kidnapping to Minnesota, life there after our relocation. This is just as essential as paying the bills, doing the laundry, cooking, cleaning. Taking care of myself—doing this soul work—is an adult activity, even though it is not often named as such in our culture. I have always been one to go against the grain. My novel and the family secrets it breaks are just one of many examples. Upsetting the familial ethos invites anger and fear and grief to surface, lies to tumble, secrets to bleed. But I chose this. Adulthood is meant for breaking down barriers. I used to think being an adult meant being able to compete in a world that judges me by my social status, my career, how much money I make, how articulate I am, how well I can market myself. That is all bullshit. What matters is only how authentic I can be. The rest be damned.

Sadness is present today. Smelly rubbish is surfacing from biological, subterranean landfills . . . I must learn to love it to death. Death. Death. My therapist says that my psyche is shifting. She cautions me to proceed slowly and respect myself. I must not rush. I tell myself over and over, *Sit with it. Be with it. Feel it. Trust it. It won't always be this painful.*

Chapter 2

I have been seeing a speech therapist in an effort to help alleviate my strained voice. He gave me speech lessons that include repeating vowel sounds and inserting a small rubber tube between my gums and the backside of my upper lip to stretch the tissue. He tells me that my upper lip sits too close to the tip of my nose. This adds to my speech impairment. That and my incorrect tongue placement. He gives me small, adhesive-backed, colored dots to place on my bathroom mirror and the dashboard of my car to remind me to find my "spot." This spot lies in the indentation at the roof of my mouth, in the tip of the hollow. I have been lax, letting my tongue rest behind the back of my lower teeth. This strains my tongue, which in turn strains my neck, causing tightness in my speech.

My whole body is one tense contraction. When Sarah, my Ortho-Bionomy bodyworker, tried to work on my neck, I stiffened. "Mary, what's going on?" she asked.

I told her the work reminded me of how trapped I felt when I was six years old and being sexually abused by an older male relative. Sarah asked me to explore the feeling. I started shivering. My arms and legs trembled, my knees ached. I brought them to my chest. Sarah held my hand. I felt less scared, or at least more willing to be scared.

Later that evening, heavy rains and a tumultuous thunderstorm pummeled the Twin Cities with tremendous lightning and fierce winds. It reminded me of how my body shivered its emotions onto Sarah's bodywork table. Those old, angry ghosts are foreboding, but they belong to me and I will keep trying to face them, head-on. I want to learn to befriend them, shower them with loving-kindness and compassion. My intention is not to exorcise them but to acknowledge and embrace them as part of who I am, as much a part of me as the color of my eyes or the curve of my hips, as valuable as any light and joyous heart could ever be.

My life partner Jane and I went to a friend's house for dinner. I had a nice time, even though lately I have been shunning social gatherings because it has been so difficult to talk. I am trying to get to the root of this problem, but I am not having much luck deciphering the reasons for my bizarre, strangled speech. I spend a lot of time, energy, and money on bodywork, speech therapy, mental health therapy, searching for answers. I try to accept this outlay of cash as an investment just as important as my SEP/IRA.

I won't make it to retirement age intact if I don't commit myself to healing. It's good to have the constancy of Anne, my therapist, and Sarah, my bodywork person. At least when I am with these soul-workers, I feel safe enough to admit how stuck I feel. And they don't comment about how my voice sounds, like others.

"Do you have a cold?" is a frequent question asked of me.

"No!" I want to scream in frustration. "This is just the way I sound."

I feel less crazy when I don't minimize my suffering. Maybe if I keep doing my work, my past will have its say and quiet down. Isn't that what is holding my voice hostage? I have to stop denying its impact, stop telling myself that since the abuse and trauma happened so long ago they can't be important now. I have to trust that if I make room for it, I can come to a sort of marriage between my painful past and my shining future.

Sarah says it's possible to work through these things—release the hard, old memories from my body. Someday, I'll be able to recall them as a part of me but no longer define myself by them. When I reach that point, I'll feel safer in the world, fully wounded, fully healed, with all the cuts and scars, all the beauty and joy. Everything. With no apologies.

I'm trying to not define myself by my voice or the quality of the sound it makes. I have been working subconsciously as I sleep asking Spirit to help me accept my voice with all its raspiness, its starts and stutters, its choking, halting sounds. I can note how my voice connects with what I'm feeling and try to dump all judgments, sending them to do their negative bidding elsewhere.

Even this, though, is a hope, as yet unrealized. The reality is that I haven't been reading any of my work at my writing group lately because I am afraid to read. I am afraid my voice won't work. I slip and define myself by the quality of my voice instead of just reading and not caring about what others think. Maybe I'll try to read something short next time. Give it a trial run. I can practice not judging myself and put how my voice sounds into perspective.

Chapter 3

Confidence is a sore spot for me, especially when I have to speak in public. It's as if my personal power were a raging waterfall and my audience a crowd of thirsty travelers. My power doesn't just seep out, little by little. I dole out bucketfuls to whoever is present. I replay internalized messages: *I am worthless, stupid, ugly, untalented*. These feelings crash through the floodgates and banish my courage. I have already started to worry about my reading at Odegaard's bookstore. It's nearly a month away, and I am having small panic attacks about getting up in front of people. Maybe if my voice doesn't work, I can humbly decline any future offers for readings. I'll probably not have to decline them. They won't be offered. There I go, judging myself. I want to turn it around, make how my voice sounds be okay, just the way it is. Why is that so hard?

I feel frustrated, betrayed by my own body.

Jane and I have been attending Tonglen classes facilitated by Julia, a local Buddhist teacher. Tonglen is an ancient Tibetan meditation technique that seeks to transform personal, emotional pain into compassion. The meditator inhales all that is painful, choosing to embrace it, befriend it instead of shunning it, then exhales compassion and loving-kindness toward herself and others.

All week, sadness has been roosting on my chest and in my gut—old war-horse grief. At meditation on Thursday, my heart expanded for a brief flash of time. During that session, I experienced an awareness so deep I felt it on a physical level. Somehow I understood, in the pit of my heart, that *No Matter What* is essential in my current struggles with my writer's voice, my physical voice. Writing that novel was like breathing in the dark, rough, hot, hard emotions—fear, anger, grief, sadness, impatience, rage (as one does when one is practicing Tonglen) and breathing out loving-kindness, the gentle acceptance that everyone in the world is intimately linked with these very human, vulnerable emotions.

Our Tonglen instructor said that we must learn to see our suffering as blessings. Our lessons come in many ways. Suffering can be a teacher. Our pain, our longing, whatever unnerves us, these arrive in our lives like an old friend, knocking on the door, asking us to open up. Surprisingly, what steps over the threshold is not an enemy, but a friend—in the guise of Bodhichitta, wisdom, love, and compassion for ourselves and for others.

I think about embracing the rough, hot anger that was muzzled in me as a child. It has a stronghold on my psyche and my voice. It's not good to silence the children. We need them for their wisdom. We need them for their intuitive knowing, their love and honesty. They are the way-showers. We adults try oh-so-hard to be sane and rational and left-brained logical about our goals, our purposes, our responsibilities, but we have cut ourselves off. How can we write an accurate story without reliable sources? My anger is one of the most reliable resources I know. So is my fear.

"Where there is fear, there is power," Starhawk wrote in her novel, *The Fifth Sacred Thing*. I've been thinking about that statement and about fear and the power behind it. If I let fear overtake me, it can crush me, bring me to my knees. If I rein fear in, I can tap it, like hydroelectric power. If I use it to intimidate, I can crush others. That's the part of fear that I have experienced—the inner and outer forces crushing me. But what about the empowering element? How do I get beyond the red-hot hard feelings? How do I ride my fear into another dimension and see what power lies there?

Especially when I feel that I am broken.

That is the sharpest, most singular image I have of myself as a child. Although in myriad old black-and-white photographs my bones seem intact, beneath the muscle and T-shirts, behind the massive shock of wild brown hair and the endless sadness of my dark brown eyes, my bones are fractured into millions of splinters of rage and loss.

I keep trying to touch the raw places inside. I need to gather up those fractured pieces of my soul—cull through the rubble and retrieve a slice of fibula here, a shard of collarbone there, and piece myself back together. I need to heal that which has long remained untouchable. I need my therapist, Anne, to guide me, stay with me. I need to make things right by me. Forgive myself. Stop judging my worth, my anger, and my fear. Stop labeling myself defective, broken. Stop living my life for my mother or my family. It's *my* art. It's *my* book. I wrote it for me. I had a right to do that. I had a right to my vision, my voice—both literally and artistically.

When I felt terror as a child, I didn't understand that I wasn't crazy or weird or silly. The most benign things would trigger panic attacks. When I lay in bed at night, I'd "hear" Cousin Itt from the TV show *The Addams Family* walking up the steps to my bedroom door. Sometimes I'd "see" a swarm of insects flying toward me from the shadowy corner of my bedroom ceiling. In neither instance did I know that these things couldn't hurt me because they weren't "real." They were real to me. So was the fear they roused.

More and more I am coming to understand the connections between fear and anger and grief. My voice problem won't heal until I have reassembled the fossils of my past. Even with all the speech therapy, I think this is true. The speech therapy has helped me focus and gain more vocal confidence, but the emotional psychotherapy work with Anne has helped, too. When I am feeling sadness, grief, unexpressed anger/rage, the emotions literally get stuck in my throat.

The faceless, defective, broken child I used to be, who still haunts my soul, wants her voice back. And her long bones, her metatarsals, her sacrum, her eyes, her ears, her mouth, her nose. She's been living in a world of sensory deprivation with no way to express her rage and her loneliness. She is angry and frightened. She needs to scream. She is mute yet quivering with the desire to *express* herself. This week I made a drawing of this faceless child. I gave her back her eyes, her nose, her ears, her mouth, her bones, and her muscles so she can tell her story. Maybe now she will give me back my voice. It is she who has held it hostage. Somehow, she has found a way to disable my adult self, silence her as she was silenced.

The Odegaard's reading is over. And I must honestly say it was mixed. I never felt so confident going into a reading, but my voice tightened anyway. I spiraled into a fearful, shameful place. Down and down I sank, until I could barely pull the words from my clenched vocal cords. In the end, I felt exposed, wounded, humiliated.

Jane's perspective is different. She said my voice wasn't tight throughout the entire reading. She said that I did a good job. My reading held people's attention. I hope so. I do believe that there was a whole different version of reality going on that had nothing to do with my shame and fear. I will try to trust that some people didn't judge me as inadequate because my voice wasn't crystal clear.

Doing this reading took enormous courage, and I literally and figuratively rose to the occasion. It will be hard to read my work for as long as it is hard to do so. That's the truth of it. I need only decide if I want to continue putting myself out there— exposing my naked soul to the public eye. I don't think I'm completely ready.

I did everything I could to prepare and focus for this reading, but when I stood before the audience, my conscious mind no longer had control. I fell into that familiar dark place where I lose ground. I tried to bring myself back. I made eye contact with a woman in the front who seemed to be listening intently. I stared at a row of books in the back of the room. I held tightly to the stone and the piece of bark I had placed in my hand to comfort me. I tried to breathe. Sometimes I was able to come back into my body and speak without the tightness. Other times, my voice withheld. I was able to read clearly about forty percent of the time. I guess that's a sort of success.

Later in the week, at my therapy session, I told Anne that I didn't want to do any more public readings until my voice fully returns. It drags me into that dark abyss. I end up dangling out in front of the audience. I go through the motions. I clutch for something to anchor me, something that will tether me to my stronger self, help me through, but I am not able to gain a sufficient stronghold.

Anne supported my decision. She affirmed that most people are permitted to do their healing with a therapist in private—not in public with an audience.

I need to feel my way through the emotional landscape of this journey. Somehow, that faceless child I drew holds the map. Even though I possess the conscious adult courage, the faceless child knows the path by heart. She will lead the way through and out and into healing. My adult self can't will it to be done. I have to *feel* it. And that means trusting that faceless child. For now, that means no more readings.

I feel extremely relieved.

I talked with my friend Karen yesterday about opening to the deeper pain as a way to move through it and release it. Great depths of sorrow bring great depths of joy. We talked about how some people shrink from the shadow side, fear to come too close. But the shadow is where my journey is leading me.

Speaking becomes harder and harder. It seems as if all the work I have done in speech therapy was for naught. The emotional component of my speech impediment strong-arms the physical aspects. I am trying to accept the way my voice sounds, but it is still difficult.

Is my voice my teacher? Will the tightness refuse to go away until I accept its knowledge? And what is that knowledge? Perhaps, once the lesson is learned, it won't matter how I sound. Maybe it's not about fixing. Maybe I'm not broken. Maybe this whole ordeal is about opening and accepting. I struggle to see this trial not as a pain in the ass, but as an opportunity to grow and learn more about compassion for myself and for others.

Does what I feel about my voice affect my art? Does it hold me back? Keep me from risking? There is a part of me that fears that somehow the writing caused my voice problems. I dug too deeply, excavating unhealed grief, unutterable pain. I should have left things alone. I should have written about dolphins or taxi drivers—anything else. Ironically, when I was writing my novel, I felt whole, alive, and vibrant.

In my kinder moments, I understand that *No Matter What* was something I had to "get down," as Cameron says in *The Artist's Way*. Art is not about making things up; it's about getting things down. What I create is part of me and part of something else that is not me. *No Matter What* rushed out of me, poured itself onto the computer screen. It had a reason, a life, a purpose of its own.

Somehow the urge to break the silence prevailed. The art was born, my physical voice was entombed. Why? I wish I knew. I keep writing and sculpting, drawing and praying to find out. Last week, I drew a picture of a daughter trapped inside her mother. Then I drew a picture of a daughter with her head emerging from her mother's chest. And another with the mother cocked open at the waist, a hinged box, revealing the daughter's body trapped inside. And one with the mother eating the daughter, as if she were roadkill.

Can this pain be a tool? Is it the compost, the fertilizer that feeds the rest of me? This stuff about my mother is scary. I have a deep longing for a mother—for *my mother*, or at least for the mother I wished she had been able to be. I can hardly feel what those words mean. I know they are true, this insatiable ache, this well that never fills, this emptiness that cries from a place ancient and brittle.

My mother always said, "I love you." She freely dispensed hugs and kisses, but somehow these displays of affection became chains, not wings. Knowingly or not, my mother used them to enslave me, not empower me. She was a woman of stifled passions and thwarted ambitions. Forced to give up her dream of marrying her first love because he was neither Italian nor Catholic, she was also pressured to abort her hopes of becoming an actress. She settled for a life she did not want and marriage to my father, a man she did not love. Too many children and not enough money fueled their incessant bickering. With no foundation of mutual trust and respect the marriage was doomed. The tension mounted. Her despair spiraled, creating an emotional war zone for all of us. Finally her extramarital affair sealed our fate. There may have been hope for my family if Mom had been able to learn how to love my father or if Dad had been able to be more present, less a victim to his own secret wounds. Damaged souls, every one of us. Damage to the Spirit is passed on, as surely as eye color and blood type.

Hugs and kisses aren't enough to nurture a soul. Constancy. Safety. Independence. These fuel the flight of powerful wings.

Chapter 4

In meditation class today, we listened to a cassette tape of a lecture given by the Tibetan Buddhist nun, Pema Chödrön. Pema spoke about a man, recovering from physical and sexual abuse, who used an image of caged birds in his meditation. In thinking about what image I could use to release my childhood wounds, the metaphor of a birth canal arose. The daughter trapped inside the mother, in my drawings, bursts forth with power and might and pain. Mother and daughter alike feel the struggle of the birthing. The struggle of separation, individuation is not clean or easy. The mother can't give birth without acknowledging that what once lived within her now breathes its own air, fills its own skin, cries its own cries.

Drawing the picture of my daughter-self escaping from the mother has freed something in me, something intangible, yet real. Things are moving—shifting psychically. My voice struggles are connected to the unholy trinity: Grief, Rage, Shame. Do I learn to recognize the warning signs, learn to work my "program" and stay clear of the dark, unhealed places where the demons dwell? Or do I unlock that deep terrible place and invite the demons to brunch? They are part of the family. They are way-showers. They help me know when I've strayed from the path of self-nurturing, when I'm in perilous territory. They are not Other. They are all parts of me, all my precious "kids." I must learn to love each of them—unconditionally.

Anne finished reading *No Matter What* and recommended that I consider not seeing my mother for a period of time in order to give myself enough emotional space to safely complete my healing. Her comments frightened me. She even said she'd call my mother to tell her not to contact me and that if Mom had any questions she could call Anne and talk with her on the phone or come in for a therapy session and see Anne in person.

As Anne talked, I fidgeted in my chair. I looked at the floor, out the window, at the wall to avoid eye contact with her. She noted my anxiety and withdrew her request. She said that her primary concern was that I find a way to protect myself from my mother's manipulation as I continue to work through my childhood memories. She asked me to consciously do something to protect myself before I return my mother's phone calls or before I spend time with her in person.

My mother's face haunted my mind. I could see her crying as I told her I couldn't, wouldn't see her any more. I could feel my stomach tightening, knowing I had failed to be a *good daughter,* a loving human being. Suddenly, the cold reality of my relationship with my mother hit hard. I could smell it. Taste it. Touch it. All denial was erased. Even in my hour of need I put her needs first.

Later at home, my rage simmered. How can I extradite myself from the life-sentence of being the doting daughter, the self-less one? How do I quell this deep yearning for a mother who understands that a daughter has needs, too; the kind of mother that my own mother can never be? How do I feel the loss without getting swallowed whole by it? As a child, I needed my mother as much as I needed air and water. She wasn't consistent in her giving. There were many times when her own pain and losses prevented her from acknowledging my needs and my pain. The emotional ground she provided was shaky, but it was the only reality I knew. When she couldn't meet my needs, I bided my time until the next hug, the next *I love you* came along. I nourished myself with leftover scraps, fed right in to her unconscious ruse to have me love her so she could love herself. My memory of her as a safe cocoon is a lie. She wasn't safe at all. But I'm no longer a child. I no longer need her to feel loved and safe. If only I could let the shivering center of my heart know this.

Instead, I drown in the illusion of mother love. I spiral through thick waters, murky and muddy. In my mind's eye, I gasp for breath, swallow mouthfuls of bitter liquid. My eyes swell with toxins. My skin bloats with river soot. I sink and sink. I want to sleep, to close my mind, shut out the empty hole I fall into and into. Down and down I fall. My mother calls to me. She tries to pry open my mouth, push air into my closed lungs. She wants to give me life. Resuscitate me. She tells me, "I gave you life."

I sink deeper into the river of memory to escape my debt. I clench my jaw. My top teeth puncture my lower lip. I push my tongue against the roof of my mouth so I do not have to swallow her air. Her chemical spill, her oil spill, her radiation love that slithers to catch me. I swim through the murky wet and push my arms against her chest. I kick my feet against her belly. Out. I want out. Let me drown. Death is more inviting than the sweet breath she tempts me with. She grabs at me. Her fingernails scrape my wrist. Blood rises and clots. My skin refuses to open to her greediness. My hair tangles around my throat. It wraps long tendrils around my mouth, creating a jail she cannot open. My kidneys tighten and shut down. My heart slows. My lungs close. My brain numbs. My eyes refuse the light. My ears swallow water. They fill and fill with silence. My nostrils pinch, protecting me from the threat of her. My fingers no longer sense temperature. I am not cold. I am not hot. I am not feeling. I am a mass of inert gases. A mass of explosive defiance. I am a child taking back her only power: *the power to refuse to cooperate, the power to refuse to breathe.*

I dreamt that I'd been transferred to a new high school during my senior year, and I didn't know any one. The school had many rules and regulations, and I wasn't happy. Those restrictions went contrary to my nature. My mother didn't arrive until after the graduation ceremony, and then she left quickly, saying she had something else to do.

The day before that dream, I'd struggled with low-grade sadness. Perhaps the dream was my way of releasing that emotion. Always this sadness about my mother, this longing for what never was, for what can never be. In Buddhist teachings, it's the longing, the attachment that jails me. However, it's not easy to detach. I must try to let myself feel the yearning, not make it an aversion —that, too, is a way to detach. I must learn to embrace it and go into it, not run away from it. So easy to write. So hard to do.

I dreamt last night that I was in Seneca Falls, my hometown, for a big family reunion. There wasn't enough food for everyone. I felt very upset and responsible.

Today, I feel as if writing *No Matter What* was the ultimate act of treason toward my mother and the ultimate act of liberation toward myself. I experienced this sense of freedom once before when I came out as a lesbian. And again when I decided not to visit my mother ten years ago, the first time I was in therapy with Rosemary, my former therapist. There is something strong and powerful inside me that allows me to commit these rebellious acts. Some sort of will to live and to thrive. Something spiritual and whole and divine.

I begin today with this offering: *May my heart be open and receptive.*

I had a reading by a student who is in an advanced class taught by Jane's psychic teacher, Ruth.

She told me that my Second Chakra contains a chain that links me—back through many generations—to all the women in my family. I stand at the end of this chain. The last link is broken, and I am holding onto each of the open ends, trying to decide whether to close them and become the next link in the chain or to be a pioneer and forge a different link.

The student said that my Third Chakra was fluid, much joy about the work I'm doing and the process I'm undergoing.

My Fourth Chakra (Heart Chakra) held much emotion. The student said she sensed it "exploding with feelings." She told me that I have a tendency to splat my emotions. She said that I needed to learn to work with my feelings and let people help me get at what's behind them.

In my Fifth Chakra (Throat Chakra), she saw an image of me shouting. People were passing me by, ignoring my cries. Ruth stopped by for a moment, to check on her student, and commented that my Fifth Chakra indicates that I have a hard time saying no, a hard time with conflict.

The student was unable to discern if my Sixth Chakra (Third Eye) was clear or just feigning clarity. At the Seventh Chakra, the student saw angels and music. The channel was very open. It nurtured the rest of me.

I sculpted a Spirit Child figure today. The amazing thing about her is that her mouth is *wide* open. She is shouting. She wears three scars—at her throat, her heart, her genitals—but the throat scar is open and red. The truth is seeping out.

Sometimes in my therapy sessions with Anne, I feel as if I shouldn't say what I want to say. I fear I am going to be harmed or hit for telling the truth. I am puzzled by that sense of impending violence. I woke this morning realizing that as a child I witnessed my father reprimanding my eldest brother, David, by hitting him with his belt strap. I also witnessed my mother hitting David with a hairbrush. My parents meant to scold him. He was branded a willful child. I remember my mother yelling at David and my other brothers when they would run from her.

"Take it like a man," she'd holler. "If I have to chase you it will hurt twice as bad."

It was the '50s and '60s. Spanking was permissible. Corporeal punishment was dispensed when a child failed to obey, surrender. Was it child abuse? Not by the standards of the day, but witnessing it frightened me, propelled me, even further, into my role as a *good girl*. I learned to shove my needs deeper and deeper inside. I learned to keep my mouth shut. I saw that when you sass back or defy your parents, they can hurt you.

Now, as an adult struggling to open the long-locked doors, to let in some much-needed air, it is difficult to let myself be competent, able. I shrink back. I try to be invisible. I panic. Doors and windows inside me clamp shut. My voice tightens. I can't breathe. My body cringes. As if all the cells agree, simultaneously, to stiffen.

How do I dismantle this automatic response? Doing my art forces things to loosen. I used to believe that I was safer with all these errant feelings locked away. As a child, it was probably true but not so now. I am free to choose differently. My spirit knows this. So does my heart. My cells are slower to comprehend. Physical matter transforms at a lethargic pace. My armor is thick. It exists for a reason that may or may not still be relevant. I must dissolve it slowly, carefully, respectfully. My spirit, my emotions, my body, my mind each has concerns and needs about removing the protective shield. Too often they disagree about the pacing.

My last speech therapy session is today. I am disappointed that after six months of almost weekly visits, I'm not "cured." My voice is better, but it's not 100 percent. I'm afraid my voice is never coming back. Maybe, I'm stuck with this garbled speech. No matter how hard I wish and will and want the old voice to return, it might not. It's gone. I must deal with that possibility. Even when it is difficult to do so.

I sculpted a clay figure of an archetypal mother-protector last night. I called her Crone—for her wisdom and her strength. Her face is green and brown and orange—colors of organic, growing things, colors of comfort and power, hope and redemption. Somehow, this clay figure guides me. Crone protects my unhealed Self. She is that part of me that is open and loving—and fearless enough to lick my wounds, clean them to a lasting healing. Crone helps me see that I must listen to what the hot, hurting places inside me have to say. Not run. Not hide. I choose this way. I invite these lessons. I want to traverse my path, rocky and hilly, smooth and straight, level or bumpy. It is mine.

Little by little this year, I have begun to discover that I am bolder and braver than I ever thought I could possibly be. I am a troublemaker, a boat rocker. I won't settle for lies or for the false sense of security that comes from burying dreams and stifling my heart. Every part of my adult life has been a thrust to unearth the truth of me. I *do* make waves. Not loud, crashing, attention-getting ruckus, but strong, steady, and sure, nonetheless. I rock the boat. I tip the damned thing over. I plow through the mountain. I seek change. I risk growing. I don't accept the status quo (familial or otherwise). I push the limits of self-knowledge. Always delving deeper, trying to know, to understand, and to love myself. More and more, I am discovering that I possess a quiet strength and a deep passion to push. I am BIG and I am small and I am connected to my past, my present, and my future.

The child part of my Self has wild hair and laughs—a lot. Her eyes are excited, intense, and playful. This wild child says, "Come on in, the water's fine." She tells me I am much more than my wounds. She wants to inhabit my blood and my bones, become the me I was intended to be. To assent, I must allow her to expand from the tight core of shame in which I confine her. I must allow her to stretch her cramped arms and legs so that she can grow to the edges of my skin. I wonder what will become of my voice if I can only let this child have her say?

The diaphragm-strengthening exercises that my speech therapist taught me have been helping me support my voice. The air slips more easily through my vocal cords. The words emerge with less strain. Breath empowers speech. Breath emboldens the lungs of that silenced child I once was. Still, I must be patient. For as much as the exercises have helped, my voice remains strained, resistant to returning to its former state. Easy does it. *You can't push the river*, or so the old saying goes. I might as well welcome the current, be it slow and meandering, or fast and furious. Sometimes it's both at once.

1995

Chapter 5

It's terribly cold. A high of six degrees with wind chills below zero—typical Minnesota January. I try to imagine sunshine so intense it compels me to hurry toward shade. I call forth the hot sand of July beaches. The grains burn my toes as I hop to the concession stand to buy an ice-cream cone. Sweat drips down my brow. My armpits are sticky. The skin on the back of my neck prickles from the heat.

According to my recent astrology reading, today—January 4, 1995—is the day that my old childhood and my new childhood will confront my adult self. Together, they will forge a new identity—

more authentic, more playful. What will that look like? Feel like?

I had a healing session yesterday with Ruth, Jane's psychic teacher. Ruth encouraged me to play as a way to circumvent old patterns that inhibit me. Is this a coincidence? Play was also a strong message running through my astrology chart. Is play the secret passageway? The holy road to freedom? And what does that look like? How does a forty-year-old woman play? My hula-hoops have long since disappeared. My roller skates given away to the Salvation Army, years ago. My jacks and my coloring books lost to umpteen moves and relocations.

Later, hours after my psychic reading, the energy still surged through my legs, feet, arms, and hands. I felt as if my insides had awakened from a long slumber, as if the July heat I had earlier imagined had found a way to pierce the cold ice of my resistance. Is this the way people who aren't blocked feel in their bodies, everyday? If I invite play, will this tingle of energy take up permanent residence inside my skin?

The next morning, I woke thinking about how to stop thinking and just let things happen. Progress is stifled when I shut myself into a gloomy attic of secrecy and shame. I need to open the attic door and invite my wounded child-self to inhabit the entire house. In my mind's eye, I see her faceless, mute—with no eyes, no mouth, no ears, no nose. She is a touchstone of where I have been and who I really am. My sense of playfulness was injured, this is a fact of my life. Now, as an adult, I must be fierce in protecting this child who moves through the world without her senses. I must be compassionate toward the pacing of her progress. There will be no lesser children in my household.

I dreamt that I was flying—soaring around the room, twirling in the air, making great circles, arms extended. In the dream I longed to fly through a wall. Part of me cautioned, "You can't do that" while another part of me urged, "Yes, you can!" I stuck my hand through the plaster, and the rest of me easily followed. I flew through another, thicker wall as well. My hand slipped through, then my arm, and then the rest of my body. On the other side, I kissed a woman who was washing dishes.

This week, Jane and I saw the movie *Safe Passage*. At one point, Susan Sarandon (who played the mother) was watching a videotape of a track race in which her son was competing. When he crossed the finish line, his feet didn't touch the ground. She remarked to him that he ran with no effort because he was running for sheer joy. I cried. In my life, there have been very few things that I have done for sheer joy. I try too damned hard at everything.

Once, in my twenties, I scored four goals during a single soccer game. I was able to dribble downfield and kick the ball past the goalkeeper into the waiting net. In most other games, my footwork wasn't as skillful. I was less able to dodge opponents. But that one, effortless time, my actions rose from a place of freedom. It was a glorious moment for me, not because I scored four goals, but because I was totally, purely happy. Joy fueled my accomplishments. There was no striving. Can this be what play is like for an adult?

There is no safe passage for me in therapy. Unlike that effortless soccer game, I struggle to release words from my clenched vocal cords. I can't rely on the standard, talk-therapy route. My voice doesn't hold up. So, with Anne's help, I am learning how to dialogue with my body through mindfulness, drawing, and clay sculpture. I ask my body for help in understanding what blocks it from effortlessness and pure joy. What inhibits its energy? What prevents it from flowing electric and unimpeded as it did when I scored four goals in that soccer game some twenty years ago?

My body patiently reminds me that I am merely human,

fallible, mortal. It knows my limitations. I can't fly through a wall or soar across a room. That body of light and air lives only in my dreams. In real time, my body speaks in twisted muscles. Its stifled cries are lodged in a tight diaphragm. I can't breathe. I can't speak. I panic. The anxiety is more than psychological. More than emotional or spiritual. Something clicks off, causes me to shut down. Something sucks the air out of my gut, tightening the muscles in my throat, squeezing the words out of my vocal cords.

I need a translator. Why is this so hard? What dialect am I trying to decipher? Will I recognize its cadence when I hear it? I have no control over what is happening to my body. Only knowledge, acceptance, awareness, forgiveness, tenderness, and compassion. These are my tools. These are my dictionaries, my thesaurus.

Lately, I have been feeling a deep longing that manifests as extreme hunger. I want to eat and eat and eat. It is not a physical hunger. I crave something else, some desire that I cannot identify. Last night after dinner, I decided not to give in to the food cravings. I rode out the waves of yearning, and after a while the urgency stopped.

The next day during my Ortho-Bionomy session, as Sarah worked on my neck and shoulders, I had the sense that I was young again and in the room where the sexual abuse had occurred. I saw Nate's face, so familiar to me—the young man who abused me. I saw the top of his head. I felt his weight. I tried to allow the memory to float up and wash away. I knew that, now in the bodywork room, it was Sarah who was touching my shoulder—not Nate, the relative I knew and loved, the one who had harmed me. I had the power, this time, to say "Stop!" and "No!" This time I could choose to move the energy. Memory is a kind of energy. It is cellular and psychic and stored in cytoplasm and DNA. I can let it go, too, when I am ready. It is okay to release it. It is okay to remember.

What I remember most are the bristled edges of Nate's brush cut. Like a well-loved hairbrush, turned abrasive against the tender skin of my scalp. Only, it is not my scalp that he yanks, no long brown strands of my untamed hair fall to the bedspread, floating on the quiet air like girlish wishes.

I remember the Venetian blinds, slanted against the afternoon light. The room strains for sun, aches for the day to release its longing, its fear of the dark, but the blinds remain cocked in a slant of silence. *Don't tell*, he orders. Outside, the afternoon sky blazes a glorious blue, but its color of joy is misleading. The promise of a lazy afternoon, roaming the banks of the creek with my best friend, was not to be that day.

I watch the cord swaying, the ivory bell-shaped handle hanging from the cream-colored cord, dangling from the blinds, wishing I were small enough to crawl into the cave of its opening and escape. I stare at the ceiling. Its plaster cracks suggest an alleyway, back roads to freedom if I could only move my legs, only reach my small arms, only push the bristle-headed brush cut off my sinking body.

My body goes numb. Whatever was alive and fierce slips away from my muscles and bones and hovers above the bed—watching, unable to stop what is happening. Years later, I remembered that I had no breasts. My chest was flat with six-year-old nipples. I wore a gray-and-brown sweater with fringes along the bodice, a second-hand castoff from a richer, older cousin who had outgrown her girlhood. A cousin who stood then at the edge of her own womanhood, as least as old as the bristle-headed Nate who called me into his room. *Come here. In here. Don't worry.*

Months later, on the slate sidewalk in front of my family's two-story house, Nate would steady my bike as I hopped onto the seat. His strong arms stabilized the two-wheeler, conferring a confidence I could not muster on my own. *You won't fall. You can do it.* He coached me along the blue vein of slate that led away from my doorstep. Coaxing, urging, holding, still holding until my feet pumped the pedals, and my hands anchored the white rubber handlebar grips, until I could maneuver the chrome bars, until the wind blew back the errant strands of my always-wild hair.

Without my realization, he had let go. I moved through the sunlit air, paddling on two rubber tires upstream through the river of slate sidewalk, under the power of my own legs. The same legs he had pinned to the chenille bedspread, at last pedaling away.

Later still, when he and I were years older, Nate bought a shiny, black second-hand Chevy. He washed and waxed its exterior to a bright sheen. He vacuumed its interior upholstery, its floorboards, and its rear window ledge until it was dust and dirt-free. Perfect car.

One summer afternoon, as I carried a neighbor's empty *Smith's Dairy* bottles to her front stoop for the milkman to retrieve the next day, I cavalierly swung the clear glass containers, feeling good about my charity. Too forceful in my contentedness, I hit the wooden railing, shattering the glass. Shards fell from the air like lost angels, slicing my left ankle. A lob of tissue hung from the white bone, a dainty, bloody tear.

I ran across the yard to my house yelling, "Ma! Ma!" In seconds, my mother called Nate and asked for a ride to the hospital. In the back of his beloved Chevy, I sat on the slick, vinyl seat, pressing wadded sheets of paper towels against my ankle bone to stifle the flow as the bristled brush cut cautioned, "Don't get blood on my car."

I didn't. I wouldn't. I couldn't.

I bled into the white paper towels, careful not to spill a drop on the polished interior of Nate's sanctified Chevy. Seven black stitches were all that remained of the milk bottle accident. The meaty flesh of my anklebone reconnected to its origins. Seven black stitches that mended into a pale scar. A visible reminder of how Nate had once chauffeured me to safety, even as he had, once, chauffeured me to hell.

Bodies. Shame. Breathing. My body. My shame. My breathing. My breath shallows when I feel shame. My body tenses. Silent and still. My body whispers, *If I keep quiet, they won't find me. They won't hurt me. I can be invisible. Disappear.*

Cellular suffocation. If I don't breathe deeply, I won't remember. Feelings will burrow into my cytoplasm, swim through the mitochondria, seeking hiding places. My cells won't cooperate. They command me to breathe. Every strand of DNA shouts, *Remember. Breathe from your soft belly. Pay attention. Wake up. It is time.*

I sculpted an archetype of a warrior out of modeling clay. I gave this fierce woman a red face, lightning-yellow arms, magenta legs. I placed a purple snake between her breasts and gave her a purple tongue and short black hair. Snakes appear on her legs, too—one blue, one yellow. Small red and blue circles adorn her body. Power circles. She is magnificent and courageous. Her face is kind and strong. She is, above all, tender and compassionate, loving the journey more than the outcome. When I was finished, I placed all my clay sculpture archetypes on the dining room table. I set Crone—the mother-protector—beside Imp Child and faceless child—the two clay figures that represent my wounded child self. I set Warrior to the right. I placed a candle at the top of the circle and a bowl of water at the bottom. I laid stones, bark, and my carved turtle fetishes to the left and to the right. I placed my guardian angel hanging-sculpture (a gift from Jane) above the rest. I grounded myself and cast a circle to the four directions. I stated my intention to honor where I have been and seek blessings for where I am going. I played James Taylor's "Secret O' Life" and

Sweet Honey in the Rock's "So Glad I'm Here."

I danced and sang along, "I shout out my name. I shout out my name."

I dreamt that Nate died of liver cancer. I woke up. I wonder if this was a precognitive lucid dream, or if it arose from my subconscious, as a way to tell me his power over me is dead. In the dream, I grieved for him. He was middle-aged although he was a teenager when the real-life abuse occurred. In dreamtime, he lacked the power of youth. His once-strong muscles were flaccid. He was impotent in a sense. Not at all scary. I felt no animosity, just relief that he was finally dead.

In therapy, I spent the hour listening to my body trying to better understand the places in which my shame hides. It was an exercise in being still and paying attention. I closed my eyes and felt sensations hot and tense in the pit of my heart, the core of my throat, the center of my belly, the root of my pelvis, the soul of my vagina. An image of a crumpled piece of paper arose in my mind. Anne asked if I could smooth it out. I did, and a wave of purple energy flowed up my torso. I noticed sentences written on the pages. *I am bad. I am defective. He's too heavy. I want to move. It hurts.* Anne asked if I could use the purple light to erase the words. I told her I didn't want to erase them all—just the ones that said I was broken.

Later that week, my right shoulder felt tense and tight during my Ortho-Bionomy session. I focused on that aching in a further attempt to communicate with my body. Statements raced through my head. *Leave me alone. I am not here to take care of you. I won't be taken advantage of.*

When Sarah moved from my chest and shoulders to my ears, anger and fear pressed against my skin, trying to escape. The pressure in my ears grew tighter. My legs ached and twitched. The right side of my face, near my nose, my upper lip, and my jaw, grew numb. I shivered. Sarah suggested that I turn on my side and curl up. I cried. With every breath, I shuddered.

All the restless anger I feel toward my mother and Nate is breaking loose. This problem with my voice may not be physical, but it has physical manifestations. I keep saying this over and over again, but I can't find anyone who fully understands. Except maybe Sarah and Anne. My ribs, chest, shoulder, neck, and pelvis are storehouses of fear and anger.

My mother typically chooses the serpentine method of asking for help. She doesn't just pick up the phone and say, "Something hard is going on. I need your help and support to make some changes." Being direct would go against her nature, even though it would be a refreshing change. I might very well choose to respond and offer help if she would own her feelings, take responsibility and ask for assistance. That would break our toxic pattern in which I am the initiator, the one responsible for her feelings or for pointing out how she repeatedly boxes herself into uncomfortable situations. The old way unfolds all too predictably. I confront the issues, share my concerns; she cries, but nothing changes. She accepts her predicament and I feel used, angry, and frustrated. Who is the mother here? Who the daughter?

In her audiotape "The Unmothered Child," Clarissa Pinkola Estés talks about the collapsing feeling that the unmothered child can feel in adulthood when someone challenges her or is mad at her. When this occurs, she retreats to her past wounds and acts out of that pain, without being fully conscious of the slip and without having control over the back-step. This is true of me, lately. I long to become invisible. The world isn't safe. I feel threatened and confused but it doesn't make sense on the real, physical plane. There is no actual danger to me from the people that I encounter at the grocery store, at the gas station, down the block.

Pinkola Estés notes that the unmothered child could be surrounded by people and situations that imbued love and it wouldn't be enough because what is/was missing is an essential, internal guide. This inner way-shower leads one through the journey of life and helps one to see the quagmires. It teaches a person that she is strong and capable. It helps her name her strengths and weaknesses. One's biological parents are charged with this duty. When the parents don't, or can't because they are damaged themselves, the unmothered child grows to adulthood devoid of an internal sense of safety. She lacks the ability to navigate through the rough waters of life. Hence, she has a profound hunger and loneliness that is never filled.

For the unmothered child, the challenge, as an adult, is to nurture herself and create an inner Mother Guide, such as my archetype of Crone. This is accomplished through self-care and self-love. And, Pinkola Estés adds, *you can't heal what you don't let yourself feel.* That's the hard part, the part that defies all attempts at merely intellectually understanding mother-loss. One has to grapple with the dirty mess of emotions that ensue. One has to open a vein and bleed, trusting that someone or something will be there to catch you when you swoon.

There are gifts, too, that accompany those of us who were unmothered—tremendous strength, tremendous intuition, and a tremendous power to heal.

This sadness I feel about my relationship with my mother is tangled and gnarly. I understand that intellectually. Why can't I own that in my gut? There aren't any bruises to document my traumas. No scars to point at, no physical reminders. It is easy to pretend that it didn't happen, or that it wasn't so bad. Must I learn to love that baby who is ugly and demanding and cursed beyond all recognition? Must I feed it, wash and clothe it? Take it to my breast? That babe is mine, but everything in me is repulsed by her. She is too needy. She is too weak. She is too vulnerable. She is too me.

What kind of courage can I cull from my frightened heart? What fortitude can I pump into my anemic lungs? I need to cry and to scream. *I am motherless.* Is that why I cannot speak without struggle? What has happened to my voice? Will I end up like Ada in Jane Campion's movie *The Piano*? A self-enforced mute? Will I need to become fluent in sign language so that I can communicate? Maybe then, I can escape this death of voice, this impotence of speech. Maybe then, I can fashion an alternative mother to soothe away the silence, to help me learn to live out loud.

My chest is taut; my solar plexus is tense. I've had a low-grade headache for a week. The ache presses against my temples, behind my eyes. Some dammed-up, wretched thing is poised to burst. And I don't know when or where or how it will happen. I am struggling, always struggling.

I brought old childhood pictures to a therapy session. I thought showing real images of myself might help me feel more compassionate toward the child I used to be. I have a hard time forgiving myself for being powerless and unprotected. Anne asked me to say that to the girl in the photographs. When I did, the girl I used to be defended herself. *I didn't do anything wrong.* Anne asked me to repeat those words out loud. It was difficult. My voice clenched, but I managed to pull the sentence out. Then Anne repeated my words. On the breath of her strong voice, they rang with determination and authenticity. Before the end of our session, Anne asked me to look at that picture during the week and repeat the message—*I didn't do anything wrong*—so I could begin to forgive myself. I promised to try. Retrieval work, I called it. I am a psychic archeologist, going back to excavate my lost girl soul, trying to piece together the shards of her life, the fragments that lead me deeper into this mystery.

The marketing person from my publishing house called and asked me if I'd do another reading for *No Matter What*. I told her I wasn't interested right now.

She persisted, "Why? Are you too busy?"

I lied, "Yes. I don't have the time."

I didn't tell her I was taking a break from readings because they were too hard emotionally because of my voice. I wasn't able to say that I had to make a decision to not put myself in such an exposed position until I felt ready. After I hung up, I felt guilty for saying no.

I fell on the ice and fractured the radial bone in my left arm. Getting dressed with one arm takes longer. Pulling my pants up and down to pee is a struggle. Putting on my socks and slippers is difficult, too. I have to ask for help and depend on others, even for everyday simple things like washing my hair, cutting my food, zipping my winter coat. I'm most comfortable in the role of care-giver, the one doing everything for others. It's so damned hard to have needs.

Later, when Jane washed my hair in the kitchen sink, I felt shameful and started to laugh. She asked me what was going on. I told her it was nothing, but my tears betrayed me. I sobbed as she washed and rinsed my hair, my face dampened by the mist from the faucet spray nozzle, by the wet of my own tears. I felt so damned small, so damned powerless. I felt needy even as I also felt I had no right to feel needy. What a hard place Faceless Child hides in. It is a cave of grief, dank and dim. This relentless loss curls itself around my liver, wraps its greedy fingers around my spleen. It roars and roars until I can hear nothing but my own screaming, feel nothing but my own loneliness, my own neediness come to scratch and claw at my sorry face.

My broken arm is confined to a fiberglass cast/splint. I feel caged. I want to scream, yank the thing off, flail my arms around. I want to mend this bone, soothe the fracture to wholeness. It is the same trapped feeling my body remembers from childhood. My body had a childhood, too. I forget that sometimes. It experienced the minor bumps and scrapes, the measles and mumps, the flus and other maladies of childhood. It also experienced the tension, the terror, and rage of abuse. It recorded these impressions like photographic negatives in its cellular memory. My body is a memory book of everything that has ever happened to me—good and bad.

Last week, during my Ortho-Bionomy session when Sarah gently touched my fractured radial bone, I spiraled into the all-too-familiar grief cave. This time I remembered to breathe through it, permitting the emotion to dissipate. I began to notice that my arm craved the comfort offered by Sarah's hands. She told me that she believed my arm would heal quickly—the energy in the fracture wasn't emotionally attached to the injury. My wounded bone is not the sum total of me. It would be nice to be able to apply that insight to my voice, my grief, my abuse scars—to see them as merely wounds that can heal and not as irreversible parts of my DNA.

Chapter 6

I am reading Jean Shindoa Bolen's *Crossing to Avalon.* The book tells of Shindoa Bolen's mid-life crisis and her spiritual pilgrimage to sacred sites around the world. It occurred to me that a mid-life crisis *is* a spiritual pilgrimage. One doesn't have to go to places like Chartres Cathedral or Glastonbury to encounter the sacred. One has to journey past one's personal armoring and touch the vulnerable belly of one's own Soul.

I am in the midst of my own pilgrimage. My way of perceiving myself is in flux. I am encountering one of those rare times when I am invited to know myself better, forge a stronger relationship with my psyche, and give witness to my life in ways that are mysterious and magical. It is often painful but not always. It is a time of great opening, great sensitivity. A time to listen deeply and come to trust my Self. That is the ultimate gift. Listening for my sense of the Divine, trusting that I am more than the pain of this transition.

Jane and I went to the Asian American art exhibit on exile at the Walker Art Center. Most of the work dealt with being lost to one's native culture, both by having moved away and relocating to the United States and by being Asian American and constantly being pushed toward assimilation.

The art mirrored my struggles to acclimate to Minnesota. I have always felt like a refugee here. When I first arrived as a thirteen-year old, I felt displaced. I had been taken from my Italian American roots and put in a cultural milieu that was predominantly Germanic and Scandinavian. In the two-day drive from western New York State to Minnesota, all my reference points had shattered. Set down to re-root in a land that felt foreign to me, I began the slow and tenuous process of emerging from childhood into adolescence. At the Walker Art Center Asian American exhibit, image after image reflected the quest to reclaim what had been taken. Paintings and sculptures exposed the aftermath of oppression and how it seeks to snuff the human spirit. Still, Spirit doesn't die. In the artist, Spirit re-surges in expression, in connection, in breaking silences.

This week in my therapy session, I talked with Anne about the day my mother took my sisters and myself and left my brothers and father in Seneca Falls. On that fateful afternoon, I had no power to change the course of my life. I knew my mother was going to leave, *someday,* but I was not prepared when *someday* turned into that brisk autumn afternoon. I had come home from school for lunch, and we left a half-hour later, without warning or good-byes. I felt nothing. Partly, I was numbed by the shock of actually leaving. Partly, I feared Mom wouldn't take me with her if I didn't tell her it was right to go, good to go, time to go. *Don't cry, don't make Mom feel like she made a bad choice, don't dislike my stepfather, don't say how much I miss my dad and brothers.*

During the session, Anne asked me to call on my archetypal mother image of Crone and ask for protection, so I could confront my real-life mother. I took a deep breath then spoke to the chair, imagining my mother sitting across the room from me, listening.

"Mom, the leaving hurt me," I confessed. "I'm mad at you for choosing to go in that way." I asked the imaginary chair mother why she had left my brothers behind. How could she do that? I told her I was angry that she never said she was sorry.

Later at home, I sculpted a basket out of clay and yarn and twigs to hold my hardest feelings, so I wouldn't have to store them in my chest, my belly, my throat. The emotions merged with the clay and surged through my fingers into the muddy red vessel. I felt washed clean by the messy expressions of angst. I felt listened to and heard. Accepted and soothed. Found. I felt *found.*

I have noticed that lately I have been a little less quick to judge my voice. I have tried to be aware of what sets off the strangled speech. When I feel vulnerable, my voice weakens. When I am angry and not owning it, my voice tightens. When I am not confident, it tenses, too. If I continue to work at being tender with myself, will my voice return to me in full power?

A business associate of mine drowned herself in the Mississippi River this winter. Her death reflected back to me my own raw despair, my own urge to be done with it. What made her cross the line? What compels me to hold back?

49

I am obsessed, wondering if she went to the river thinking the quiet would ease the terrible shiver in her head. A walk would be nice. Her feet would touch the ground, remind her that she was in need of comfort. Did she touch the trees as she passed? Did bony branches catch the edges of her coat, asking her to reconsider?

Thick and wet snow soaked her hair, her coat, her tired shoes. Did the water seduce her? Did she think for a moment that it would be quieter under the icy river? Did the rocks catch her eye as she fell forward? Did their cold lips kiss her face, tell her to hush, now, hush? It's over. It's over.

The current pulled her down and down and down into the river's waiting lap. She died, there, cradled in the Mississippi's murky comforts. I hope she has found peace, at last. I hope I am not seduced by the water's pull. I want to claim the river's edge, stay safe and warm on its teeming banks.

I dreamt I had to climb a towering tree to escape something that was chasing me. I climbed and climbed, finally reaching the top. The highest branch was very narrow. As I looked down and out over the horizon, I was overcome with fear. To quiet my heart, I looked to the sky. I swung my leg around the thin tree branch in order to shimmy down the other side. As I began my descent, I wrapped my arms and legs around the tree, as if I was hugging it. The tree inhaled. I could feel its breathing belly touching mine, feel its heart beat against my chest. I knew I would be safe, knew, too, that I would arrive at the place at which I was intended to arrive. The challenge is also the redemption.

Chapter 7

I was asked to do a reading at Amazon bookstore in Minneapolis as part of a celebration of National Feminist Bookstore Week this coming May. I politely declined. My voice still isn't up to it. After the phone call, I tried to read, thinking that if I sounded okay I would call back the woman from the bookstore and agree to her request. I opened *No Matter What* and read the first sentence out loud. My voice reverted to its halting cadence, its swallowed words. I couldn't articulate what I had written. I closed the book and cried.

I had a very powerful Tarot reading last night about my voice. The circle contained many potent cards—Daughters and Sons, Shamans and sixes (which, ironically, represent exuberance). The indication was toward balancing my internal male and female energies. All eleven of the cards were positive. The outcome card was the "voice card"—a stunning image of a woman's face with swoops of color rushing out of her heart and her throat. It made my heart race.

Two of my brothers and their friends made a game of taunting me when we were young. They would stand in the side-yard and yell *crybaby* at me through the open kitchen window. Inside, I would bite my lip, stare at the turquoise cupboards, and try to contain my tears. I did not want to prove them right. Some days the name-calling wasn't enough. On those occasions, my brothers and their cohorts would sing a song they had invented. In unison their voices would rise, *Let's have a cry a cry a C-R-Y/Let's have a cry, a cry, a C-R-Y/Come on Mary give us a cry.* They were merciless. Sometimes I swallowed back the tears. Other times, the hurt cut too deeply, and I ran sobbing to my mother. I wanted to claw at their mean-boy eyes, kick their evil-boy faces into the dirt. But I didn't know how. When I asked my mother to intervene, she thought, instead, to toughen me up. "Don't let them get your goat," she admonished, but she didn't teach me how to accomplish that goal. I was a shy and sensitive child, not innately mean-spirited. I did not know how to defend myself from my brothers' organized hostilities. My mother's pep talks did nothing to educate me. Instead, her advice to hide my injured heart—and not let the teasing bother me—pushed the onus of culpability onto me. My brothers' contempt became *my* problem. Something in me needed fixing. If I could only change my reaction, I would be all right. Mom never named the boys' behavior as improper. My crybaby tears were the real culprit. Shame flows naturally from such an inverted reality.

I painted watercolor images of a cupboard from a dream I recently had. I chose rich colors—yellow, blue, orange, green, black, and red. In one painting, I drew a girl's face and hands reaching for an open, but empty, cupboard. Inside, the cupboard was devoid of color, as bleak as my heart when my voice fails me.

I dreamt about rape. In most of the dream I was an adult, although my feelings were those of someone much younger. I felt vulnerable and powerless. In the beginning of the dream, a group of men were stalking women in a hospital. One man tried to be friendly, but I panicked. My intuition told me he was trouble. He grabbed me, but I freed myself and raced off to a part of the hospital that I knew would be more crowded and, thus, safer. The dream shifted to my family's old apartment in Minnesota. My writer-friend Ellie was supposed to come for an overnight, but our plans changed because of the rape epidemic. My two sisters (who were little girls in the dream) were also in the house, in their own bedroom for safety. Groups of rape survivors came to my door asking to be let in and cared for. I joined Ellie at a rape crisis meeting to discuss what to do about the situation.

I went to the movies with a friend to see "Dolores Claibourne." It is a psychological thriller as well as a study of class and emotional/sexual abuse. The movie is a treatise on the Good Mother. Dolores does what she does in order to save her daughter from incest. It is a parable about patriarchy and women's place in it. The daughter is estranged from her mother. Both women are victims of the same man and of the same culture that seeks to silence them. In the end, Dolores's daughter returns home to help her mother during a court trial in which Dolores is accused of murdering her husband. A guilty verdict would surely result in her being sent to prison and maybe even executed. Dolores had killed her husband in order to save her daughter from further abuse. By the final scene, tension still exists between mother and daughter, but there is reconciliation, as well.

The sexual-abuse element of the movie was difficult for me to watch. I closed my eyes, but I heard enough to make my stomach turn and my vagina tighten. I sat still and quiet. My breathing grew shallow. Sweat dampened my upper lip. I tried not to listen, tried not to spiral into my own abuse memories. It felt real. It felt *very* real.

That rape dream I'd had a few nights earlier dovetailed with what I was witnessing and hearing on the movie screen. All week, I hadn't been able to shake the shame and anger and grief. I felt crazy harboring feelings over something that happened to me thirty-four years ago, but it can still undo me. I tell myself that I am being too sensitive, letting it all affect me—like I did the cry-baby taunting of my brothers and their friends. It is hard to hang on to my right to feel angry.

In 1987, I sent a letter to Nate. I told him that I remembered that he had molested me when I was a kid. I told him I was putting the responsibility back on his shoulders—where it belonged. I had carried the shame far too long, thinking the abuse had somehow been my fault. In writing that letter, I named the truth and reclaimed a piece of my life. I took back my power, as therapists would say, and maybe they are right. I admitted, for the first time, to the person who had harmed me, that the abuse hurt me. As much as my mind tried to minimize the significance of the abuse, my body wouldn't let me forget. Writing that letter to Nate made me somehow bigger than the six-year-old he had injured—even if just a little bit. The part of me that was ready and willing to speak my truth took its first, wobbly baby steps on the long road to healing.

54

I was a first grader when the sexual abuse started. Nate was barely in high school, as troubled and rageful about his life as I was about mine. He thrust his anger, his sorrow, and his confusion onto my body. We were both kids—wounded and young with torn hearts and bleary futures—this I understand now, as an adult. I also know this: whether or not he meant to harm me is irrelevant. He did harm me. And he harmed himself, too. Although my mind can barely remember the details of his actions, my body has perfect recall. It remembers the fear and the longing to push him off me. It remembers the terror of wandering for years with no connection to my own soul. It remembers its smallness—and its courage. My body was caught in something neither Nate nor I could name or prevent. We were two lost youngsters, playing out the terrible truths of power corrupted, anger misplaced. We were both casualties of a war zone that claimed us, although his age, gender, and family ties endowed him with the power to dominate and control. He stole my innocence. His betrayal broke my heart and maimed my childhood.

Writing to Nate back in 1987 wasn't the end of my healing process, merely the beginning. There is still so much more work to do, so many unclaimed parts of my soul that scream to be retrieved. Watching a movie scene can trigger unconscious memories. Reading a poem or hearing another woman's abuse story can send me spiraling, as well. Making love can be scary, too. I sometimes have to will myself to stay present, traverse the curves of my now adult body, in order to embrace and receive, give and enjoy tender touches with my lover.

Sending a letter was not enough to liberate me from the memories. What will it take to live seamlessly inside my own skin? In therapy, I talked with Anne about needing to forgive myself for being too little to prevent the abuse, too vulnerable to save myself. Sometimes, I can approximate absolution. Most of the time, I cannot.

Chapter 8

Jane and I went to Sedona, Arizona, in May. We joined Jane's psychic teacher, Ruth, and some of her other students on a five-day excursion. I was excited to go on the trip but also apprehensive about meeting new people. I was worried about my voice. Would it work? Would it be clear and strong? Or would I struggle and sputter, trying to frame even the most simple of sentences? I tried to assure myself that it didn't matter how I sounded. In the end, I wasn't convinced.

The energy vibrating off Sedona's red rock formations was electric. I felt as if someone had plugged me into a massive outlet.

A current coursed through my hands and arms, my feet and legs. We ate a picnic supper at Bell Rock. After we finished, we took a short hike. As we climbed, I felt my chest muscles ease and relax, as if my heart had grown more spacious. The rock's energy flowed through me—a circuit of earth and blood and bone. The air was thick with it. I could have dived in.

The following morning, we climbed off-trail at Cathedral Rock. The route was very rugged, the terrain was oftentimes steep, and we had to crawl over rocks and shrubs to arrive at our destination. We climbed up and up into a remote crevice. We crossed through a stone archway and entered an enclosed area, surrounded by red rocks. Interior walls rose upward to kiss a cloudless, brilliant sky. I climbed into a vaginal slit of red sandstone and azure sky, a stone crotch, carved by the wind and the rain and the snow. I felt cradled by the splendid energy, at rest in the lap of the Ancient Mother. I shivered and cried. Too long had I been separated from this most holy embrace.

Later, we removed our shoes and socks, and stood barefooted, warm skin against the cool clay ground. Thus planted, we breathed deeply. Ruth explained that we had crossed into a different time dimension. As we passed through the stone archway, we had stepped into another world. She reminded us that birds and the wind accept who they are without questioning whether they are good enough. Rocks don't desire to be birds, she told us. They accept their nature. They are honest and open and reveal who they are without hiding. They never whimper, "Don't touch me here, I am ugly."

After our communal meditation, Ruth worked with each of us individually, near a stone archway. She touched the middle of my forehead and then my neck, asking me to open my throat, to let the wind blow through. The wind swirled around me.

"The wind likes you, Mary," Ruth said. "You used to ride the wind. Do you remember?"

My heart ached; I held back tears, thinking of my clenched vocal cords, my strangled speech. She continued, encouraging me to let the wind move through my throat. She blessed me saying, "Sing your song, Mary. And let the wind carry it into the world."

When I rejoined the group the urge to weep stuck in my chest. I moved away from the others and let go of my sorrow. I cried until there were no more tears in me.

The next morning, we climbed Fays Arch in the rain. It fell steadily for hours; even though I wore rain gear, my lower legs were soaked from rubbing against the sagebrush and cacti as we hiked. My gloves, shoes, and socks were drenched. I shivered with chill.

A fellow hiker who had been leading up to that point asked me if I wanted to take over. My immediate reaction was to refuse her offer. I surprised myself when I managed a resolute, "Whoop!" The rock's energy pulled me toward the arch high above our starting point. When I reached the top I let out a *Yes!* A group member far below responded in kind. My heart leapt at the sound of us. I felt brave and capable, courageous and joyous.

Rain fell around us, but we were safe, under the protective covering of Fays Arch, tucked into the lap of the Mesa. I tried to ground myself, pulling energy from the earth far below, but it wasn't enough to warm me. Ruth instructed us to ask for guidance in opening any doors inside us that still remained closed. She implored us to identify those places in ourselves that needed healing.

I focused on my neck and my pelvis. Something shifted in my throat. Grief welled up and out. I let it tumble down the side of the rock into the canyon far below. Tears rose and fell, rose and fell. A river of loss surged from my pelvis through my torso and out of my throat. I heaved years and long memories of grief, into the rain, washing it out of my body, letting it stumble over the edge of the cliff wall. I felt released and very tired, very cold.

The following morning, we hiked Boynton Canyon, one of the most powerful of the Sedona vortexes. Again, rain fell as we left our parked cars. As we walked, it poured steadily for a long while. When we arrived at the Petroglyph turnoff, the sun broke through the clouds. We stopped to peel off layers, happy for the sudden break in the weather. Under a clearing sky, we hiked through forests peppered with oak, maple, and fir trees. Along the way, we briefly gathered near a pine tree, attracted to its gnarled branches that reached out to us like hungry fingers, groping.

During my stay in Sedona, the edges of people, trees, furniture, rocks became crisper, cleaner, more luminous, as if a veil of not-knowing had gradually lifted. Our trek through Boynton Canyon took us through what Ruth described as time dimensions. As I passed through one such time doorway deep in the woods, I sensed a coven of women chanting. I felt the shifts in the other portals on a more physical level. One time, my body suddenly began to itch. Another time, the air grew thicker, more dense, making it difficult to breathe. Still, other times my arms and legs tingled. When we reached the end of the canyon, we climbed a difficult uphill path and were greeted by a massive rock with red sandstone breasts and a large, kind face. Mother Crone. I smiled and breathed deeply and easily.

We hiked past the Mother rock, to higher ground. The rain began to fall again. We trekked higher still, until the sides of the red cliffs became dangerously slippery. Without warning, the sky plummeted us with hail. Dime-sized cubes of ice collected in yucca plants creating spiny snow cones. We retreated to a lower level to meditate in safety.

On that hillside in Boynton Canyon, I felt at home in my body—for the first time in my adult life, maybe for the first time since I was six years old. Something deeply ancient, older and wiser than I was, cradled my weariness, freeing me to release the familiar clenching. There was nothing that I needed to cling to that day on that cliffside, under the stormy Arizona sky. My arms and legs relaxed, my pelvis softened, my stomach floated on a sea of ease and something else—maybe love, or what lies beneath love, that unconditional acceptance of things as they are.

More than anything else, the striving stopped—that ever-present, ever-insistent urge to push harder, be more, be better, forget, deny, bury the tense, hard memories that burrow deep into my cells. That day in Boynton Canyon, I was five years old again, before the abuse, before the hard years of my parents' marriage had settled into permanent encampments in my bones. I was light and wholly without worry or fear, or dread.

My body became mine once more—no longer hostage to external forces. It was mine. All *mine*. And that was a most amazing sensation.

Jane and I returned home from our Sedona trip, happy to see our garden, our house. Still, I felt a strain of sadness in leaving the Southwest. I missed the mesas, the sagebrush, the juniper, the pinions, the adobe, the Russian Olive trees along the creek. Back in Minneapolis—the land of thick humidity, lakes and rolling, green hills—my challenge was to integrate the feelings I had claimed in Sedona into my daily life in Minnesota. To take the transformation and know it *here*.

In Arizona, Ruth had talked about how emotional, physical, and sexual abuse can throw people off their timing. Her words reminded me to respect my body's pacing. If I let it, it will lead me to its own healing.

Painting and sculpting connect me to my body. Writing feels less visceral lately, even though I know my writing has had its share of bodily impact.

When I create images, I don't think. I *feel*. I sink my fingers into wet clay, and my heart follows. I squeeze, shape, caress. I mold the clay until a face emerges. An arm. A leg. A mouth. Open and wide. Clay mouth. Screaming mouth. With clear emotions, I ride the landscape of my psyche. Anger. Rage. Grief. Love. Longing. Dirty hands. Clay-packed fingernails. Messy. Juicy. I wet the sponge. Water washes the thirsty clay. Living clay. Heart clay. Dirty, messy life of clay. Warriors of clay. Crones of clay. Faceless children, crying in clay. Wounded women wailing in clay. Grateful journeyers reveling in clay. Figures born in clay. Strong. Essential. Real. I am a woman creating. I emanate from the clay. I am the clay.

Is writing like meditation? Am I decoding the hieroglyphics of me? Is there a purpose to this? Or is it futility?

Writing *No Matter What* and promoting it through public readings transported me back, literally and figuratively, to my childhood. I tapped into a deep, unexplored reservoir. I told the truth about trying to survive. Now I spend a lot of time cleaning up the mess of it, the feeling and the physical fall-out that ensued. I continue to do retrieval work. Continue to exorcise my demons.

It is extremely hard work. I fall apart at times, my emotions triggered by stress or my perception of other people's expectations of me—real or imagined. My palms and underarms sweat. I fear having to be right or have an opinion. I cringe at the thought of opening my mouth to speak. Is my tense voice a manifestation of post-traumatic stress syndrome?

Post. As in after-the-fact. *Traumatic.* As in my family's brand of craziness. *Stress.* As in tense heart, clenching vocal cords, churning stomach. *Disorder.* As in lack of control, powerless to alter.

I dreamt that I needed to hold onto my Soul and not give myself away at any price.

My dad and his wife are visiting us in Minneapolis. Last night after supper, Dad shared stories about his relatives and about his boyhood in Castellaneta, in southern Italy. He talked about his life as a young man in Seneca Falls, New York. He talked about organizing a union at Gould's Pumps, a manufacturing plant where he worked for fifty years. He reminisced about his thirty-four-year career as a Town Trustee and County Supervisor, fighting for other people's rights. My father feeds us story after story—details of things I knew only superficially when I was young.

As a child, I was angry that my father could not see what my mother's affair was doing to our family. Why didn't he stop it? Now, when he tells stories of his life, I think about the things I *could* have learned from him. Feistiness. Courage to face things and fight for justice. And yet, he didn't fight for Mom. Maybe he realized that was one battle he couldn't win. He took an honorable route. He raised my youngest sister as his own without question, for five years before my mother left him, taking his two biological daughters with her. I am beginning to see my father in a different light. Perhaps he is a gentle-hearted warrior.

In my therapy session this week, I told Anne that I felt as if I metaphorically needed to murder my mother. A deep grief gripped me all day afterwards. That night, I dreamt about being in a family but not feeling as if I fit in. Toward the end of the dream, I left the fold. I finally realized that I didn't belong there. I cried because I was an outsider, but I knew leaving was the right decision.

The following week, I told Anne I was afraid that if I told the truth, the BIG TRUTH—how it felt to be abused, how it felt to be smothered, how it felt to have my essence sucked dry—then I would lose my mother. I sobbed.

I am easily irritated these days. I feel self-protective. All the wounded parts of me are screeching out of tune like a wayward orchestra. I feel exposed, which manifests as impatience, crabbiness, and anger. I get miffed at Jane for small things, nuances really, that I interpret as her impatience with or judgment of me. I feel as if I don't have a right to my bad moods. Jane becomes the brunt of my anger at times, anger that is misdirected, because she is a safe person with whom I can practice these awkward new feelings. At those times, I know I am not easy to live with. My mood changes without notice. I am bitchier and that is not behavior she or I are used to from me. Underneath lives fear. If I let myself be a bear, Jane will become disgusted, impatient, and unhappy. She will leave me—either figuratively or literally.

These demons are inhibiting my ability to function. Simple things, such as interacting with people at the grocery store, are extremely stressful. These benign encounters trigger intense anxiety. My voice tightens. My blood pressure rises. My heart races. Some noose of memory that I cannot shake strangles me. A hot coil of panic burns my throat. My voice tenses. Terror rises. It is a terror I have felt before. I am a child of six, of seven, enduring nights of bedcovers over my head, fingers in my ears in order to still the war inside my head, invite sleep to claim me. I am a bedwetter. I am a young girl escaping my body so I don't have to taste the fear, swallow the shame, and remember Nate's body heavy on mine. I can't breathe. I can't move. I can't speak. "Help!" I want to yell. "Get me out of here." No one hears. Words jolt against my clenched jaw, ricochet down the back of my throat.

Jane and I saw the documentary, *A Litany for Survival: The Life of Audre Lorde* at the Walter Art Center. This film chronicles her experience with breast cancer and her life as a lesbian, feminist, poet/writer.

Toward the end of her life, illness had changed Lorde's speaking voice. The film revealed a woman whose once-powerful, resounding voice had been diminished to a squeaky ghost of itself. When I first heard her speak, on film, my face reddened with shame. In spite of that discomfort, I somehow managed to watch how Lorde dealt with her situation. She admitted that it was hard to have her voice change, as she'd relied on it her entire artistic life to get her message out. Nonetheless, she accepted it. What else could she do? She was a warrior. And warriors endure.

I know, first-hand, that it is difficult to have a voice disability in a world that values articulation and clear speech. It is even more so because I am a professional communicator. The irony is not lost on me. It is a struggle to make my way in this speech-valuing world. People make comments, *Oh, do you ever have a bad cold.* They feel free to say whatever they want, as if they are the first to discover and identify my abnormality. I don't need it pointed out. I know intimately that my voice sounds different from what people expect. My challenge is to befriend this different-ness, to take charge of the situation. I want to boldly say, "No I don't have a cold. This is the way my voice sounds"—without excuses, without putting my emotional tail between my legs and skulking off.

Anne talked with me about doing bodywork to consciously parallel and support the work we do in our psychotherapy sessions. She suggested this as a way to help move what's ready to be moved in my body. She told me that I could stay with Sarah, my current bodyworker. If I preferred, she could refer me to one of the bodyworkers in her Hakomi group.

My body shouted, *Oh no! The gig's up!*

Anne explained that Hakomi integrates emotional work with hands-on bodywork. It is a mindful way to pay attention to the body and to one's states of consciousness. I told Anne that I needed more specific information about how this technique blended the emotional with the physical. Bodywork is an extremely intimate experience. The practitioner touches not only the physical body, but the client's history/experience as it is stored in the body's cellular memory banks. The skin is the brain, the brain is the heart, the heart is the soul. Bodywork can be extremely loaded, especially when you add an emotional/therapeutic component.

Anne told me that Hakomi is meant to help a client move blocks in those places in her body where she holds tension, fear, pain, trauma—places that are ready, willing, and able to move. In theory, the purpose is not to have an emotional meltdown but to give permission to and provide a vehicle of support for the body to release old, unhelpful patterns in a safe environment. It sounds like the next step.

Heaven help me.

Chapter 9

I dreamt I was hiding in a basement. I did this to let a team of bodyworkers know how traumatizing my sexual abuse experience was. The bodyworkers assured me that I definitely needed help. They conducted a preliminary assessment. Then I went upstairs to work with an older woman. She helped me with the more emotionally difficult pieces.

I watched a PBS special called "The Language of Life" in which Bill Moyers interviewed poets Shandra McPherson and Linda McCarriston at a biennial poetry festival in Waterloo, New Jersey.

McCarriston's story touched me. Her father physically and sexually abused her and her mother, and physically abused her brother. The poetry in McCarriston's book *Eva Mary* deals with those experiences.

In the interview, McCarriston talked about needing to write her poems in order to heal. Poetry, she said, gave her a language and a voice for talking about what happened to her and her family. Poetry helped her turn "an indignity into indignation."

Art can transform a victim status into a thing of power, a thing of anger at the violation. It is a powerful way to hold others accountable. McCarriston wrote the rawness of her experience to give voice to the not-so-uncommon experience of childhood abuse. She broke silence, and therefore, she broke shame.

She talked about how her poems were hard to write and hard to read in public. Somehow, she manages to do it, even as I cannot. McCarriston's words gave me courage. Her story affirmed that my need to write *No Matter What* was, and remains, valid. I write what I write to stay sane, to heal, to tell a story that deserves telling, to give voice to those parts of myself that most need a voice, those places that are unable to talk any other way. Suffering has its price, but healing repays the debt.

I dreamt that my mother told me she was leaving my stepfather. I said I thought it was a good idea, but that I didn't believe she'd follow through with it. She expressed concern that my stepfather would fall apart if she left him. The dream shifted. I stood on a staircase, leading to a courtroom. I was in the building to witness my mother's divorce proceedings. I passed a ten-year-old girl who also stood on the steps. She appeared withdrawn, sad, afraid. The girl was at the courthouse in connection with a child abuse/custody case. After I woke up, I realized that the child was me.

Lots of dreams last night. I was definitely verbal in them—shouting, complaining, and voicing opinions. I don't recall the context. Just this insistence that I speak.

I had dinner at my mother's house. It's hard for me to see Mom and my stepfather with my sister Teresa. Their interactions appear so effortless. Part of me is happy that the three of them have that kind of connection. Part of me is sad that I am not included. My relationships with Mom and my stepfather are fraught with landmines. I have to keep my distance, at least until I get my bearings again. It is the price we three pay for the history we share.

It's been a long time since I've done any clay or painting. Or creative writing. The very raw places are too scary to touch. I trust that the art will return. Until then, I need to tend this garden of old scars. It's in grave disrepair, thick with brambles and weeds, overgrown and unruly. If I prune away the dead excess, I will begin to reclaim the edges of my skin. I will make way for the singing and the sighing of my bones. Then my muscles will heave their weariness into the wind. I want to dance, if I can still remember how to dance. I need my body. Every cell, every sense, every bump and bruise, every wound belongs to me. Imperfect and tender, strong and resilient, it's mine. It's mine. *I haven't forgotten everything.* And I can remember the rest, if I try hard enough and listen long enough and let myself cry enough.

I may be little, but I am not dead. Yet.

Part of reclaiming my blood and bones lies in confronting my mother. What would the warrior in me say about that? *Tell your mother, You are my mother and I love you, but I do not owe you my soul.* To me, this warrior would say, *You are strong enough now. Trust in what you need. Take care of yourself. Your mother is not capable of helping you. If she were, you wouldn't be in this spot right now. Grieve your losses. Speak your truth. Your mother can no longer hurt you.*

I am a grown woman now, out of my mother's care, away from her house. I want to find a way to love her *and* myself. To do so, I need to continue to delve into the muck and the mess. It takes great courage to live life with an open heart—to not shrink from human suffering, one's own or others'. I pray that I have what it takes to see me through to the end. It's a blessing to acknowledge one's limitations as well as one's strengths. Sharing my story through writing and art is not a defect—it is an invitation to live life out loud, and not retreat.

Chapter 10

Today is my first Hakomi bodywork session. I've been waiting a long time for this piece to be presented to me. Even so, my body is fearful of letting go of its armor, frightened that there will be nothing to protect my vulnerable core if my muscles don't follow through on their job of being tense and holding everything together. I need to understand that I don't have to make my body a perpetual sentinel. I need to try to resurrect the effortlessness that I felt on that cliffside in Boynton Canyon.

I'm afraid my speech won't cooperate when I have to confess to Beth, the bodyworker, that my voice hasn't been working for nearly two and a half years. Yet, that's part of why I am seeing this woman. Will she understand that my body is the record of my living? Each cell has its own pattern, history, shape, and response to past traumas. Each must be shown a way to let that go.

Beth told me that the purpose of this type of healing work is to respect and listen to the body. To learn and accept its pace. She talked about her role as facilitator and told me that she is charged with creating a safe space. Oftentimes, clients come in expecting to work on a particular issue or body area and the body directs the work in an entirely different direction. The prime objective is to trust my body's innate wisdom. It knows exactly what it needs and how it wants to proceed. Our job, she told me, is to be attentive.

I told Beth that it feels as if there is another heart inside the hot, dense core of my body. It contains the real me, the woman that I might have become had the abuse never occurred. I touch that place when I do my art, when I connect with something greater than the pain, greater than the perimeters of my fearful, angry, grief-stricken limitations. I visit it when I let myself laugh and play.

I left the Hakomi session feeling a bit more hopeful. Beth seems to be a fine person. Maybe I can learn to trust her. She has kind eyes. Time will tell. For now, I am beginning to understand that I am changing in deep ways that I can barely articulate. Small outposts of rebels have laid down their protective armor and have opened to the clay play, the writing, and the creative visualization I do with Anne. Some of the rebels have rejoined the Union.

I heard a story once about a group of hikers on a trip in southern Colorado who used llamas to haul their gear. As they led the llamas down the trail, the animals would stop from time to time and refuse to budge. The hikers tried to tug on their leads, but the llamas stood their ground. It was no use cajoling them.

The llamas insisted on being met on their terms. The only way to move them was to stay by their sides and walk along with them. The hikers had to acquiesce to the animals before they would go forward. Like those llamas, my body must dictate this path on which I now find myself. My ego must acquiesce for my healing to progress.

Jane told me about *Art as A Way of Knowing,* a book she had come across in the Shambhala catalog. Pat Allen, the author, sees art-making as spiritual communion with one's deepest self. She talks about how to use image-making to discover who you really are inside, behind the armor, the baggage, the persona.

I think Allen and I speak the same language. When I hold clay in my hands, energy pulses between my heart and my fingertips. The energy is physical, tangible, but it is also emotional. It's the place where the two merge. There's no conflict, no shutting down physically when I work the clay. Instead, a broadening of my safety zone occurs. I create a breathing space that is free of tension and of thought. Something heals in that dimension; slowly, in small, exuberant ways the wounds suture and the scar tissue builds a bridge from past to present, from inner self to outer world.

In reading Allen's book, I feel as if I'm having a conversation with someone who truly understands that art is a way to dialogue with the body. She writes about working with intention and attention. She asks, *Where in your body do you connect with the process?*

I sculpted an altarpiece, a sacred place for my Hakomi process to begin. I placed pussy willows on the altar for softness. I added a nautilus-chambered shell to invoke transformation. I placed sage upon the clay altar for purification. I added a small stone with a pink interior to represent the womb/vagina, and a labrys to symbolize a Warrior woman's strength. I set a small clay body upon a bed of straw for comfort and protection.

I made clay Archangels—Grief, Anger, Shame, and Fear—to serve as guardians. They ensure that the Hakomi process will respect my body's needs, not my ego's. As I fashioned the Archangel Fear, anxiety bristled in my belly. My heart sped. My breath quickened. My hands shook. *Safe. You are safe,* I told my body. I set the clay down, took a deeper breath. The physical sensations lessened. I painted Fear's spear. A sentence raced through my brain: *Fear will blow your head off.* I left part of the Archangel's skull exposed, revealing a shiny silvery brain beneath its bones.

During my Hakomi session this week, Beth started working at my head and moved down to my neck and shoulder. Her touch felt safe until she placed her hand on my stomach. Fear surged in my belly, but I couldn't tell her. Perhaps Beth sensed the change. "Is it okay for me to touch your stomach?" she asked. I somehow found the courage to say, "No." Without hesitation, Beth removed her hand.

I took a deep breath, then placed my own hand onto my stomach. Beth noted my action and mentioned it out loud. I bolted upright. I couldn't look at her or tell her what was happening to me, how I was spiraling into wordlessness, into the shame of having been "caught" tending to my need for comfort.

Beth rubbed my back, assuring me that it was okay to touch my own body. I rolled onto my side. Beth asked if it was okay for her to continue with the bodywork. I nodded, and she massaged my ribs. Somehow, I found the courage to tell her that I felt cautious of her touch, as if my tissues were checking out her hands, asking, *Is she safe? Can I trust her?*

Beth said that this was an appropriate response; my body was smart to question the touch. She assured me that no one was going to take away my body's protection. She would respect what my body needed and go slowly or stop, if I needed to stop.

Later at home, my shame taunted, *If you feel the rage, the grief, the fear, you will die. If you let yourself know how scared you are, you won't be able to stay in your body. And where will you go? If you let yourself know how alone and abandoned you feel, how will you be able to go to school in the morning? Or eat breakfast? Or wash the dishes? Or kiss your mother good-bye as you head outside to play with your friends? If you let yourself know how rageful you feel, you may burn the house down. Then where will you and your family be? Out on the street. And it will be your fault.*

Later that week I sat cross-legged on the floor during my psychotherapy session, showing Anne my clay Archangels. I unconsciously pushed the heel of my right foot into the floor of my pelvis, trying to contain my emotions. I tugged at my fingers, my hands, my toes. My solar plexus tightened. My vagina clenched. My distress rose. I rubbed my face, my temples, my brow, trying to cope. I wanted to smash everything in sight, stand up, scream, run out the door. Or disappear. It took all the courage I could muster to sit through the rest of the session.

To quell my rising anxiety and help me cope, Anne suggested that I remove the Archangels. I pushed them aside, and then she used a chime bar to clear out their energy. The air lightened. I took a deep breath. I felt an urge to touch Anne's hand, to make a physical connection, but I held back, too ashamed to allow my fingers to reach out for hers. Instead, I wrapped my arms around my ribcage and closed my eyes.

Anne asked me if I could return the clay body to the altar. I blurted, "No!" I couldn't abide touching the figurine—the sculpted image of the vulnerable little girl I used to be, still was.

Anne asked if I could hold the clay figure in my hands. "No!" I asserted, feeling guilty for not loving myself enough to offer comfort. Still trying to assuage my discomfort, Anne asked if she could hold the clay child. "It deserves comfort," she said. My guts screamed, *No way. It doesn't deserve anything!* I opened my eyes, glanced at Anne's face to see if she was sincere, then turned away. Finally, I gave in. "Only if I don't have to watch," I said.

I shut my eyes as she reached for the figurine. When I reopened them, Anne was cradling the small clay body in the palm of her hand. Something deep inside me envied that creature of clay, lying where I wanted to be, in the comfort of my therapist's warm palm. I swallowed back tears as Anne offered to keep the clay child with her until our next session. It would be safer there, I told myself. It would receive the care and attention it needed, the care and attention I knew I was not ready to give it.

In an active imagination session, an image arose of a fierce mother chasing her daughter with a huge knife. The daughter ran in fear and disbelief, trying to escape, but she wasn't fast enough. The mother grabbed her daughter's hair, pulled her to the ground, and slit her throat. The daughter lay limp, oozing blood. The mother set her weapon aside and dived into her daughter's neck. Blood dripped from the mother's mouth. In her dying stupor, the daughter groped for the weapon, but she was too weak to grasp it. The daughter called upon Spirit, who rose from the daughter's body, grabbed the knife, and severed the mother's head. Then Spirit cradled the daughter, carrying her to safety. She tended to the daughter's wounded throat and gave her strong teas to build her strength. She wove strains of energy around the daughter, covered the daughter with a blanket of stars and rocked her to sleep. When the daughter awakened, her throat was healed.

In my Hakomi session this week Beth worked on my throat and talked about softening from the inside out. I cried. I tried to imagine releasing the sadness into the Pacific Ocean so it could dissipate. Instead of a dispersing wave, my mind held a gigantic block of ice. Beth suggested I try to let the ice drop into the water, giving it back to the sea.

Toward the end of our session, I was aware of energy and movement in my torso, an unexpected spaciousness. The tension in my organs began to soften. Beth told me that my body was capable of recalling this feeling. "It's like remembering the smell of a rose or the taste of an apple," she said. "You can ask your body to remember this softness, and it will."

It is easier to talk about having a body with Beth than with Anne. I am readily overcome with shame when Anne asks me where the tension arises in my body or what hurts when I have a body memory. I try to speak but I can't. The internal pressure cooker pumps away, building tension, pushing against my temples, my diaphragm, my chest. What is it that trembles so?

Maybe I need to start in the present tense. I can talk with Anne about my relationship with my body today, at the age of forty, and then work backwards. Trying to start at age five or six is too difficult. Maybe I can tell Anne what I do like about having a body. My body serves its purpose. It physically gets me from point A to point B. It enables me to run, garden, and walk, to feel sun on my skin, cool breezes on a steaming day. It enables me to laugh. And give and receive affection. I like touch.

What about sex?

That's a harder question. When I'm in a good place, emotionally, I enjoy sex. Even at my most centered times, however, it can be hard for me. When I am making love I feel overly self-conscious. I vigilantly attend to what is happening. I stiffen and sometimes shut down, willing myself to continue in the name of intimacy, trying for myself and for my relationship. Jane is respectful. She gently asks me if I am okay. How can I tell her that my body fears being hurt?

I can barely admit that to myself.

Chapter 11

Beth is the fourth person I've gone to for help who has told me to *play*. She said she had a sense that I work too hard. She remarked that this is a common response from adults who were abused as children. They had to grow up fast and learn to take care of themselves. This is true for me. Survival took everything my small body could give. So, I'm here, almost forty-one years later, grappling with the aftershocks. I have a body that is a work-horse, in dire need of softening. Beth and I decided to make at least part of each Hakomi session be about play.

Maybe she is my play mentor.

When I am in an Hakomi session, I trust Beth's touch. With Anne, it's different. Physical proscriptions are present in psychotherapy. Boundaries prevail, and I find myself trapped in an old definition of therapy. You go and you talk. You don't touch. Why is this so? Because of my voice problem, I've had to relinquish those old rules to a point. I can't speak very well, and so mere talking is out of the question. I've had to rely on art, visualization, and journaling to convey to Anne what is going on with me. Lately, I have needed more. I have wanted to touch Anne, have her touch me back, but I am afraid of it. Even as I want it, I am repelled by my own need. I am afraid that it is silly and wrong. Is this crazy?

Anne and I hug at the end of each session, but at that point I am no longer the defenseless young child. I am an adult again, and it's not the same. I need to touch her hand when I'm my smallest self so that a physical bridge can occur. Maybe I'm bordering on the taboo, but I feel a pull to break through the disconnection—my sea of shame—to know that Anne isn't going to abandon me. None of this can be resolved unless and until I talk with Anne about this issue, I know, but I cringe at the thought of revealing this to her.

During our session last week, I finally managed to broach this touch thing. After much stammering on my part, and an insistent urge to look everywhere in Anne's office except into her eyes, I confessed. Anne was unruffled. She told me that she had used therapeutic touch with clients for many years. She holds and rocks some clients; others she just sits next to or reads stories to or holds their hands. I told her the thought of her holding and rocking me was unsettling. That kind of comfort felt way too intimate. I said I could envision touching her hand or having her put her arms around my shoulders. She said that was okay with her. I felt relieved. I wasn't crazy. This touch thing wasn't off the wall. She hadn't tossed me out of the room for being despicable, too needy.

I have run too long and too hard, trying to escape the difficult, messy feelings. And my uneasiness at wanting to be touched by my therapist is one of the messiest yet. There must be something in me that will benefit from my need for physical comfort from Anne.

I want to free the wild shame-child that romps through my heart. I think that's possible, but it takes believing in the power of witness and emotions. It takes me being willing to trust Anne and trust my own shaky needs. If I am to survive this journey, I must allow that child to hold my therapist's hand until she no longer needs to.

These past few months, I have been in a highly contractive state—withdrawing, protecting. In September, I will travel to northern Minnesota for a writing retreat at Norcroft. This impending sojourn is an important piece. Norcroft represents a place in which I can rest and restore myself. I've been so exhausted from work and the therapy and bodywork. A break will be good.

I crave the solitude and the quiet beauty of the North Shore in autumn. Autumn is my season. The time of my birth, the anniversary of our leaving Seneca Falls, the season in which my first novel was published. It is a time of great pain and sorrow as well as a time of celebration and joy.

I will be one of four writers-in-residence. Living with three strangers is not going to be easy. My fears about my voice are high. It's been two years since *No Matter What* came out. Still, I continue to struggle with my speech and the resulting issues of exposure that my writing entails. Still, I continue to grapple with the importance of writing and art in my life. Still, I cringe when

I am asked to read my work out loud.

It is difficult to love my ugliness, to accept my limitations. Maybe I should write myself a permission slip to be scared, to be excited, to be compassionate, to have a different voice, to be wounded. Give myself permission to be who and what and how I am. Give myself permission to risk things and to change my mind about risking things. Give myself permission to accept and open to this gift of time that Norcroft brings. Let it help heal me in any way it can.

In preparation for Norcroft, I have packed cookies and Earl Grey tea, so I can enjoy a midday repast in my writer's shed. I've packed my art supplies and a few CDs, so I can feed my soul. I've packed running gear so I can feed my body. I've packed a camper's chair, so I can nurture my need for rest and contemplation by Lake Superior. The road up north, the road inward, the road outward again, these things I will know more about by the end of September.

Chapter 12

It is beautiful here at Norcroft. The property is set back from the highway on a heavily wooded lot abutting a rocky shoreline. There are two big buildings—one large main house for the writing residents and a smaller, separate one for the caretaker. Five small writing studios (which they call sheds) are situated on various parts of the property a short walk from the main house.

The residents' house is open and spacious. A large living room/dining area and a mammoth stone fireplace occupy most of the first floor. The kitchen is roomy and stocked with goodies. Residents can write requests on a chalkboard in the pantry, and our caretaker gladly obliges us on her bi-weekly grocery shopping excursions.

My bedroom (named in honor of Audre Lorde!) is situated off the living area on the main floor. An east window faces Lake Superior. A writing desk sits near the quilt-covered bed; shelves of books await perusal. My writing shed is nestled in the woods. Trees surround me as I write, in a studio named for Zora Neale Hurston.

I slept long and well in my Norcroft bed. Slowly, in this place of quiet and contemplation, I am shedding the stress that has accumulated over the past year. Yesterday, one of my fellow writing residents mentioned that she had a hard day remembering the death of her lover eight years ago. She told herself she could make a conscious choice to do her grieving through a ritual or through writing a story. She chose the ritual. I immediately chastised myself. *You should take care of your grieving in rituals instead.* Later, it occurred to me that the woman's choice to do a ritual over writing a story denied me, and others, the chance to learn something about grief and what it means to be fully human. Of course, the woman had every right to choose the ritual over the writing, but I needed that counterbalance thought to realize that my choice was equally valid.

Interacting with the other residents is easier, more spacious, than I imagined it would be. Everyone seems equally enthralled with this gift we have been given. The generosity is returned in open hearts, in laughter, and in the sharing of community and of writing. As this first week unfolds, I am losing track of the days. I am disconnecting from my city life. I do my best to trust that whatever is, is, and to accept each day and what it brings with the intention of inviting compassion to greet whatever arises.

The Tibetan Buddhist nun, Pema Chödrön, says that our spiritual journey consists of everyday experiences. The hard stuff counts, too. It's not about reaching some peaceful place of bliss and staying there. It's about staying present and waking up each moment, to the good and the not so good.

I spent the day on a huge boulder, just offshore at the Lutsen Resort. I nestled into its sturdy lap and watched the lake. The sun glistened on the water. I had a heart-to-heart chat with the Mother of all Lakes—Superior. A friend once told me that she believed Superior is big enough to hold any sorrow. I confided to the Lake that I was tired of struggling. I longed to be happy, to feel safe in the world, to feel as if I belonged. I cried a deep cry, then watched Superior's slate-gray waters lap gently against the perimeters of my rock fortress.

I have completed a workable draft of my new book, *A Talk with the Moon*. I now have a fairly tight manuscript, thanks to these days at Norcroft. At last my memoir collection of essays about my relationship with my father hangs together as one cohesive story. Time and attention are what it needed.

Even as I finish, I've been obsessing, again. What will my father think about these essays? What will others read into them? Do I care? I write what I write to understand my own process of healing and reveal the truth of what people endure in families. Pain and sorrow touch our lives in different ways, but this is what unites us as humans. Suffering is something we all share in one form or another. To transform it, we must find the hidden jewels in the dirty muck, the treasure in the dark cave of our sorrows.

I woke this morning with an idea of how to craft a sequel to *No Matter What*. I had struggled with whether or not to even attempt such a project, even though people who had read my first book urged me to do so. I was insistent that no sequel would be born unless I could figure out a way for the protagonist, ten-year-old Peanut/Regina, to be healed or at least be given the tools to eventually do so. That key transformative piece was missing in the chapters I had been able to draft before I arrived at Norcroft. Now, a way has been given to me, a way that makes sense and is also interesting enough to develop into compelling fiction. Peanut would have to encounter an alternative mother figure, someone who could nurture her enough to give her hope, inspire her to love herself, against the odds.

Tomorrow marks the end of my second week at Norcroft. Tonight some of my fellow residents are planning to read their work out loud. I am trying to trust my heart and not be swayed by peer pressure. I am going to delay my decision as to whether or not I should participate, until later this evening. I don't want to ruin my day obsessing about it. I also want to be free to make a decision from the present moment, as much as possible, assessing how I feel about reading out loud, when we gather together, instead of basing my choice on whatever fears I may be feeling beforehand. If I feel safe enough later to risk it, okay. If not, I'll decline and give myself permission to do what is best for me. I want to be able to offer compassion to myself in whatever ways I can, regardless of whether I choose to read or not. I want to approach this decision not as good or bad, as success or failure, but as an indication of what I am feeling in the moment about this particular voice, free of judgment, free of shame.

Today is September 30th—the twenty-eighth anniversary of the day my mother, sisters, and I left my dad and my four brothers.

I want to do a ritual to help release the impact that this experience has had on my life. If I continue to memorialize this every year, perhaps, little by little, I will begin to soften the hardness, invite other possibilities, know myself as more than just that terrorized girl who lost her daddy. I need to remember *I can choose joy*. Here's to growth and to healing, to the splendid waves of Lake Superior, and the deeply sacred woods around my shed.

Today will also be my last full day at Norcroft. This tremendous gift will feed me for quite a long time. I have experienced joy and belonging, creativity and peace, loneliness and fear, anxiety and grief. I am learning more about how to love my inner demons. What you resist, persists, someone once said.

It's true. It's true. It's true.

Chapter 13

I am in transition from the solitude and quiet of my writing retreat to the din of Duluth—a small port city, south of Lutsen. Built in and among the hills rising above Lake Superior, Duluth is lovely and quite manageable as cities go; however, being in an urban setting once more feels odd, after the peace of Norcroft. I hope I can, in some small way, hold onto the gifts of slowing down and listening that I found in my North Shore writing shed. Norcroft is in my bones, and I must make time for the things that sustain me—my writing, my artwork, my spiritual practice.

Jane took a bus from Minneapolis to Duluth to spend the

weekend with me before we drive back to the Twin Cities together in my car. We haven't seen one another in three weeks, so it is good to spend time enjoying the outdoors and each other. One day we hiked the east section of Gooseberry State Park. The afternoon was foggy and overcast, creating a stunning backdrop for the muted oranges and yellows of the trees, the reds of the rock lichen, the golden moss and grasses. The colors were breathtakingly rich against wet, dark rocks.

Later that night as we made love, a deep sob unexpectedly erupted from me. I cried hard for a long time. I felt as if my body had cracked open and wrenching loss spilled out—uncontrolled and uncontrollable. The sob rose from the socket of my pelvis and surged through my chest, up my throat, and out of my mouth in a rush so powerful I couldn't catch my breath. As the grief crested, joy followed. In the aftermath, I felt completely open, fully connected to my muscles and my bones. The next day I felt awkward. I wanted to shield myself from such perfect intimacy.

Back in Minneapolis, I find it hard to settle into my life without my Norcroft writing shed, without the sacred space carved out each day for my work. I know it will take time before it feels natural once more to look out my window at busy Bryant Avenue, let the roar of city buses wash over me until they become just background music to my daily comings and goings. In Minneapolis, there is no commanding lake as mammoth as Lake Superior, but there is Lake Harriet three blocks from my house and numerous other, small city lakes with places to walk and think and be. The challenge is to let the healing unfold, no matter where I find myself. My path is peppered with interior landscapes.

I have been writing again, working on a sequel to *No Matter What*. I'm in the dump-and-run, first-draft mode, but that's the beauty of it. The story spills out uncensored from the expanse of my heart. Then, when the passion and the energy are recorded, I go back and polish it. The writing keeps me sane, offers an outlet, a way for me to communicate without my speaking voice. I can shout and rant, cry and laugh, celebrate and enunciate all that is in my soul without ever uttering a single word.

During my Hakomi session this week, my body began releasing layers of tension. When Beth worked on my ribs and under my shoulders, energy flowed from my feet through my chest and arms. My body felt more spacious and strong; as if my insides had been shaken out, like a dirty rug.

I started taking Calm Spirit tablets this week. I wanted to experiment with whether they could help reduce the anxiety that fills my days. If they do, I plan to start taking them regularly. Maybe I have a chemical imbalance. These pills are not a magic bullet, but if they help ease my day-to-day functioning, along with psychotherapy and Hakomi, then they are worth a try. I also decided that it's time to focus on my neck and throat in my body-work sessions. I want to explore the emotional ghosts that are locked inside those parts of my body. What's inhibiting my voice? I want to release it.

I am beginning to understand that what I fear most is not *outside* me. My body is a scrapbook of all my experiences. Recorded forever? Perhaps. But maybe, just maybe, the memories can fade, like old pictures.

I wept throughout my Hakomi session. I felt defective. I felt angry, sad, fearful. It's so difficult to have my body's reaction to its past abuse be so visible. Others can hear my struggles in my voice. I am exposed. And utterly alone.

It is hard to function as a capable adult when I cannot speak.

I deeply want someone to help me, to heal me, to take my hand and lead me through this hell. But I am afraid to ask. It's hard to trust that anyone would want to walk this perilous road with me.

What I want most is peace. If my voice is going to be a permanent physical change then I need to grow into acceptance. Surrender is difficult. Maybe that is the bigger picture, the reason for this journey—to learn how to love myself, with all my wounds.

I confessed to my friends Patti and Karen about my voice struggles. They know I have been having a hard time talking. They have heard the strangled vowels, the mangled consonants, but I have never officially talked with them about what is happening to my voice. I felt scared, but I am glad I finally opened up. I need to come out of the closet, so to speak. I allowed myself to be honest with two friends whom I trust. Both Patti and Karen are capable of witnessing pain without trying to fix it. Nothing is more sacred than that. The more I can let down my guard, the better I will be able to embrace a peaceful acceptance of my voice—the way it is.

I am learning that befriending painful memories requires immense stamina. Healing is fraught with labor pains, back pain, pushing and shouting of all manner and kind. It is a thing of blood and guts, a thing not for the faint of heart.

One of the things that impedes my progress is my strong visceral reaction to being the center of attention. Am I re-experiencing some ancient trauma? Or is the shutting down a stop-gate to prevent me from remembering? And what am I trying to forget? I feel such hot panic. My insides prickle with anxiety. I feel the urge to curl into a fetal position. I want to pry back my skin, escape this burning building of bones and muscle. There is a little kid trapped inside me, and she has a big mouth. She wants to yell, "No!"

I never got mad as a kid. I couldn't afford to. Anger would have alienated my mother, driven away the one person who felt safe to me. I invested considerable energy in being a *good girl*. I never complained, never sassed back, never said, "I don't want to." As an adult, this acquiescence has come back to haunt me.

Whether I retrieve my voice or not, acceptance will come only if I steel myself against the challenges and call on my courage. Then, the old, greedy-fingered grief and fear can abate. I will someday know that these murky emotions are not the entirety of me. At the core, I am gifted and compassionate, brave and confident, ready and able to speak my truth, trust my place in the world.

I dreamt I was back at Norcroft. Large groups of people were there, including Jane and my sister Teresa. We attended workshops, and we drew pictures to depict our personal stories. I drew a picture of Regina, the ten-year-old main character in my novels. She was bathed in yellow light.

It snowed last night. A light dusting of white coats the trees, the ground, a silent harbinger of winter. How I hate the cold and the length of it. How I hate the darkness. The 5:05 p.m. sunsets, the 7 a.m. sunrises. The bone-chilling freeze that descends upon us up here in the northern lands. I've already begun to wear layers of clothes and wool sweaters.

We spent Halloween at Ruby and Cara's house again—passing out candy to hordes of goblin-clad children. I love Halloween. Once a year Death/Shadow throws a party, and everybody celebrates. The envelope between this world and the next is explored, accepted, and invited in. And I can attempt a kind of truce with what is unseen, learn to trust my own ghosts and all that dwells beyond the realms of what we call reality in our day-to-day lives.

As the cold, dark months of winter close in, I worry that Death and Shadow will linger too long in my house. I have been tired lately, depressed, and emotionally spent. I've been meditating the last few days for twenty to thirty-minute stretches. It has helped me slow down and realize that I can create safe spaces inside myself when I need to.

But will it be enough?

Chapter 14

My voice has been extremely tense lately. At supper one night, I told Jane that I couldn't converse with her. It made no sense to strain. Doing so would only make my voice worse. I decided to honor my body and trust that I needed to be silent. I didn't try to figure it out intellectually. I accepted it without shame or anger. Big lesson.

During my psychotherapy session this week, I had an abuse flashback. I couldn't breathe. The room grew smaller. I wanted to shrink, to be invisible, slip away, escape from the walls that closed in on me. I told Anne that I felt as if I were being set on fire.

Inside, the panic boiled. My body felt as if it were being pressed against a wall or pinned to a bed. Was it Nate? Or my own panic that smothered me?

Scorching energy smoldered inside me. I could have burst into flames. My body twitched, anxious to escape. I sobbed, grieving for my body and the abuse it had endured. As a child, I didn't know how to make myself safe. My arms and legs were not strong enough to push Nate away. With no hope of getting free, my body switched off. Some part of me hovered above the bed, witnessing the horror as it transpired. How hard it has been to forgive my body for not being able to flee. As an adult, I struggle to find ways to reclaim my bones, to comfort my aching heart. Anne asked me to place my hands on my body and offer it solace.

"I'm sorry for abandoning you," I whispered to my legs. "Sorry for leaving you to fend for yourself," I whispered to my belly. In tears, I repented to my pelvis, my chest, my legs, my arms. As a child, I didn't know how to help them escape. Now I do.

For days after therapy, I have felt weepy. I cry at the least provocation. I sob over a sappy tune about new worlds and new possibilities I hear on the radio, from the Disney movie *Aladdin*. I'm tired of this struggle. I want it to end. I took Jane to work one morning, and when I was driving home, I thought about taking pills or maybe jumping off a bridge. To let go of this world like my colleague had done a few years before. What would it feel like to be in mid-air knowing I was going to die as soon as I hit the water? Would it be freeing? Would it be a great rush of release to know I never had to struggle again? Or would it be frightening? Would it fill me with panic and dread and the shocking truth that I couldn't go back, like a cartoon character changing direction in mid-flight. Would it horrify me that I couldn't change my mind and grasp for the ledge, safe again on the hillside?

Lately, I have been a prisoner to my own struggles. I want to be fearless, but courage has been sorely absent. It has been a hard week for my voice, too. No doubt the coincidence is not coincidental. I haven't been breathing well, and I feel small and powerless. Some part of me knows that fighting against my voice is not the path to take. Surrender is the surest route to freedom, but I have been very attached this week. I grieve the loss of how easy it used to be to just open my mouth and take for granted that words would tumble forth clearly and unstrained.

What is snatching my breath from my belly? I am frantic. I want to crawl into a hole, bury myself and cry, cry, cry. I have been unable to get my head and my body back in synch for the entire week. Most of the time, my body operates on automatic pilot as my mind and heart wander about, disconnected from my legs and arms, my torso. I'm overcome by an unrequited longing for the reunion of my body and my soul. I feel abandoned and deserted.

Beth suggested that my body's reaction was really a demonstration of its wisdom. It knew it could not handle the trauma of remembering the abuse. Maybe my Soul and my mind opted for temporary exile so my body could process its pain, later, when I was able to be with someone who could help. Sometimes, disassociation is the smart choice. It can help slow down the process. The body really *does* know what it needs. I just have to trust it.

During my Hakomi session this week, Beth and I tried an experiment. I took a deep breath and held it as Beth gently pressed against my upper chest, saying, "Meet me. Meet me." The point was for me to expand my lungs to meet her fingers, then turn my head and exhale as she pressed against my diaphragm, helping me expel air. I took a deep breath and held it, but felt compelled to exhale swiftly—before Beth was able to say "meet me" more than twice. Panic flared. I felt trapped, then shameful and defective.

Beth explained that my diaphragm was sucking up when it is supposed to expand downward, thus leaving my voice unsupported. "You need new wiring," she told me. I laughed and suggested that we start calling our sessions a bodywork version of "This Old House."

Have we uncovered the underlying problem? Is my body/nervous system sending the wrong signals to my diaphragm? I am inverting, sucking up when I should be opening and expanding. That literally shuts off my air supply. Beth explained that everyone's body needs re-wiring somewhere. Ground zero for me just happens to be my diaphragm. She suggested I try to observe, without judging, so we can see how to work with this new information.

I suck in when I inhale, instead of expanding out. My voice is robbed of the power of my breath. Is this the physical manifestation of my emotional truth? Instead of approaching my healing with a critical attitude, wagging my finger and shouting at myself, "You're forty-one years old and you can't breathe right!"—it's more helpful to explore my body's tension with curiosity and exploration. "How is the breathing easier here? Oh, it's neutral here. It's harder there."

Charging at my body will only make it resist and revert to clenching. Breathing will help. Breathing connects me to the emotional language of my body. I need to explore it, accept it, let it speak in the ways it knows how.

Later that week, I mentioned the Hakomi breathing exercise to Anne. I described my penned-up feelings as being locked in a box. "What do you know about this box," she asked.

I started to talk, but the words stuck in my throat. Anne asked what the mute part of my child self needed to feel safer about telling. With starts and stops, struggle and frustration, I managed to reply, "Tenderness, comfort, and safe touch." Anne asked, "Do you need safe touch from someone other than Beth and Jane?"

After another fitful try, I managed to tell her, "I need safe touch from you, Anne."

Panic continues to claw its way into my Hakomi sessions. Beth touched my diaphragm with her fingertip and I cringed. I told myself, *She is safe. What would it be like to trust her? What would I see if I just explored, with curiosity, what lives under my diaphragm?*

In my mind's eye, I discovered that my diaphragm was covered with a metal grate, beneath which lay stacks of boxes and a lot of dust balls. Beth asked, "What is in the boxes?" I told her I didn't know. She removed her fingers to see if anything changed. I sighed, then suddenly felt selfconscious. "What's the selfconsciousness about, Mary?" Beth asked.

I replied, "Having a body."

"What could be the worst thing about having a body?" Beth inquired. My mind raced with unspoken answers. *Having a body that isn't allowed to say "No." Having a body whose bones rattle with rage.* I placed my hands on my diaphragm, curled my legs to my stomach and turned on my side, without a word of explanation to Beth. She touched my head and rubbed my back. An image arose of a small girl huddled among boxes. Her face and hands were dirty. Her hair was stringy. Her clothes were filthy and tattered. She was tired. And emaciated. She was me.

Touch continues to be a difficult topic in my psychotherapy sessions. We decided that Anne would move from her therapist's couch to one of the client chairs and inch that chair closer to mine. This would enable her to sit closer to me and perhaps reach out and touch my hand or my shoulder, if I needed her to or wanted her to. It amazes me that such a small gesture feels like a *big* deal for me.

I still struggle against the internal messages that this change of seating arrangements is a silly thing to need, but I agreed to try. So, when Anne moved her chair one tiny inch closer to mine, my gut screamed, *She's going to hurt me!* But Anne didn't harm me. The realization sank into my bones: *She is a safe person after all.* I cried with relief.

In Hakomi, Beth and I sat on separate, oversized rubber balls, and then I pushed against her palms with my hands while she provided resistance. I breathed in and out as I pushed. Anger rose, outrage rose, and the urge to push harder and breathe through it. I visualized shoving Nate off me. I visualized being strong enough to protect myself. I created space around and within me. I felt powerful and safe *in my body.* To my surprise, I felt giddy, and, strong—from the *inside* out.

Choosing when to be touched—emotionally, physically, or psychically—allows me to establish borders. This is important in my writing, too. I write to stay sane and to heal, to work anxiety out of my body. If others don't like my subject matter, if my family members have a hard time with my honesty and the feelings it churns in them, I say, "The grave I rob is my own." I am entitled to the story of my life. It belongs to me. I can do with it what I want.

I am learning that trust is a cellular contract, not an intellectual one. Breaking old patterns is slow. Sometimes I take one step forward and three steps back. After the giddiness of the Hakomi session, I felt deeply sad. My voice was extra tight.

Jane and I rented a limo with four friends and took a Christmas lights tour. My friend Ben and I hung our heads out the car windows and sang carols at the top of our lungs. We were unselfconsciously and deliciously passionate. Lightness is coming back to me, bit by sacred bit.

This is the hidden gift that rises out of the emotionally hard and draining work I do in therapy. I feel shame most of the time—shame at wanting physical contact, shame at asking for what I need, shame at feeling shameful. It is such a vicious cycle. Anne has been very present and compassionate, kind and attentive. Very patient. And caring. She holds the hope of lightness even when I am unable to do so. Somehow, it helps me carry on.

Everyday, I try to remind myself: *I am safe. I am safe. I am safe.* This tight fist of stomach can soften. I can breathe, breathe, breathe. I am a grown woman, now. It has become my mantra, my prayer. Why hasn't my body figured out that it is safe now? I must try to trust that this hell will not last forever, that I will not always think of it as hell. I must try to trust that I will be given what I need.

National Public Radio's program *All Things Considered* did a story on a man whose book, *The Middle Passage: White Boats, Black Cargo*, took twenty years to complete. People grew impatient, but at least one person supported the author and said, "You're not a 100-yard-dash sprinter. You're a long-distance runner. We need more long-distance runners."

On the TV news, I heard about a woman who survived a gunshot wound to the head during an airplane hijacking in 1985. She said she finally realized that her experience happened for a reason. It was a wake-up call to live her life more fully.

These unsolicited messages help me cultivate patience, acceptance, and compassion for my own long, arduous process.

1996

Chapter 15

My second-grade teacher, Miss Lacey, celebrated each of her students' birthdays by standing the honoree on top of her desk as the entire class sang "Happy Birthday." In October, when it was my turn, I climbed on top of the smooth, wooden surface of her desk and looked down, shyly, at my shoe laces until Miss Lacey put her arm around my shoulder, coaxing me to gaze out over my classmates. As their squeaky, off-tune voices rose in unison, my hesitancy dissolved. I stood, proudly, on top of my teacher's desk and beamed. That experience nurtured a sense of birthday entitlement in me that I possess to this very day.

The image of myself as a second-grader soaking up the celebratory voices of my classmates resides in sharp contrast to my sense of myself one short year earlier. In the first grade, the covert effects of sexual abuse caught the attention of a different teacher, Sister Saint Frances. I was quiet in class, withdrawn. I did okay on tests, but when Sister asked me to respond to her questions about the alphabet or arithmetic, I bit my lip, stared at the floor, and didn't say a word. Nothing she did could convince me to venture out of my safe cocoon of silence. I stood resolute, exuding *I-want-to-be-invisible* energy. Sensing something was awry in my six-year-old world, my teacher asked my mother if I had an inferiority complex.

In therapy, I imagined a dialogue between me as a first-grader and me as a second-grader. The two little girls stood face to face. Every time I began to identify with myself as a second-grader, feeling entitled and happy, soaking up the cheerful voices of my classmates, shame bristled. The first-grader's fearful energy overtook me, insisting that the second-grader had no right to be so bold.

As an adult, how do I make more room for the second-grader in my life without exiling the first-grader from my heart? How do I hold these diametrically opposed images as if they were twin souls of the same girl? Of me?

I am a failure if I measure my life by my mother's rules and the rules of our shared Italian American culture. I seek separation. She seeks inclusion. I seek to walk my path. She seeks to have me phone her, see her, be her partner in this emotional tango. To my mother, family is *everything*. This is incongruous, I know, given the fact that she left her marriage and her sons, yet it is true. It matters little that her choices took her outside the bounds of what was right and proper. La Famiglia demands unwavering allegiance, even from a prodigal daughter. What better way for my mother to repair the damage, re-assert her fidelity, and reclaim some of her lost honor than to enforce the edict of loyalty, of family above all else?

This cultural ethos adds fuel to the fire of my mother's desperate longing for well-being and love, a longing that she believes can only be satisfied by her children. She measures her worth by how attentive we are to her needs. I have failed because I no longer acquiesce to the role of the doting Italian daughter, the child who gives her mother comfort and grandchildren. I started out that way, but over time, I grew to crave separation, to look beyond La Famiglia for support, acceptance, love, healing. As an adult, I am disloyal by saying my family wasn't as loving and nurturing as it pretended to be. I willingly break the rules even though, when I do, it is still hard for me to not feel guilty. Somehow, that spunky second-grader I used to be has survived, at least enough to allow me to remember that taking up space in the world, separate and apart, is not always wrong or disloyal.

How do I fuel this desire for separateness without totally severing my belongingness? How do I take leave of my bones, slip between the fractured lines of familial love gone bad? My aching breath cools the air, stings my face, tempts me with the promise of freedom. Outside my skin, I am not encumbered by blood and muscle and bone. Outside my skin, it is easier to see the separate lines of my mother's body and of my own. Her head, my hands, her feet, my belly. We are distinct continents floating in a sea of air. Out here—away from the forces of biology and destiny—there is no fear of tectonic shifts, no tidal swells threaten to blur our individual shorelines.

As any child, I began life in my mother's body. I suckled the fleshy fruit of her uterus until I was ready to swim down the narrow passage into the waiting hands of the world. We nearly died that October afternoon. The two of us nearly gave in to the urge to be done with it, as if a small part of our hearts already knew what lay ahead. But begin we did. To still her insatiable hunger, my mother snatched me back to her groping mouth. She swallowed my blood before I had a chance to feel it, hot and electric in my tiny blue veins. Apart from her, away from any attachment to my body and its history, I can trace the clear edges of my skin, finger the muscles that wrap my bones, count each separate strand, smooth or striated, that insulates my life from hers.

It is not my bones that acquiesce to her cravings. Perhaps my synapses misfire. Signaling the wrong neurons, they shoot between the eyes, leaving me for dead, a casualty of friendly fire. Or is it the atria?—those open caves of red, the slosh, slosh, slosh of ethos reverberating beat by precious beat. My rebellion rattles against the hemogoblin, inflexible as steel. How did it come to this: the daughter held hostage by her mother? Away from the internal confusion, my mind belongs to me alone.

Out beyond the longing and the unmet promises, my mother's love is a cleansing wind. My lungs swell with pure air. My legs dance with pure joy. My arms sway and gather their passion at will. My un-jailed voice sings. I say out loud: *enough!* "We are not the same," I insist, until familial ties tug me back into the forest of gnarled bloodlines, twisted expectations. Bony rocks of memory name the ache between my shoulders, the dull scream in my hips, the pounding in my pelvis.

My body knows it is a prisoner of war, captured by the ancient pact that binds mother and daughter, uterus to uterus. In my imagination, I take a knife, splice a gene, prepare the agar, carve a space for a new body. In the petri dish of my womb, I see all possibilities. This is what I want: to grow a continent of arms and legs, hearts and guts; to sculpt a mouth as wide and as deep as memory; to yell at my mother's furious, confused face: *I choose me this time. I choose me!*

My mother is both my savior and my executioner. To enforce separateness, I rarely spend time with her. I know that breaks her heart. What she doesn't know is that it breaks mine, too.

I do not know if this will ever change. I do not know if she can offer me what I need and want. My mother never reveals her real heart. She presents a hypermanic persona in order to protect herself from her sorrows and mine. I can't get close. It is unsettling to be around her for any length of time. I begin to feel as if I am not supposed to be who I truly am. Perhaps my mother does not know how to forgive herself for leaving her sons. Atonement seems to me to be a good place to start, a way to begin to accept responsibility. It's the way to heal what's hurting, but atonement lingers just beyond her reach.

Part of me understands my mother's need to cower behind her personal wounds. Oftentimes, I see my wounds as a weakness, as well. I tell myself that I have to be strong, appear as if nothing will faze me. More and more, it becomes harder and harder to achieve that masquerade. That's how it felt to do public readings for *No Matter What*. In the beginning, it was thrilling. Then, little by little, my voice refused to cooperate, and I panicked. I started to think, *Oh no. The audience can see this.* I recoiled in shame. Little by little, the grief won out. Is this how my mother experiences it, too?

I watched a TV show called *Touched by an Angel* in which a man who was dying decided to reveal a long-held family secret. He wanted to tell his son that his sister had a different biological father. The man's wife had conceived the girl during an extramarital affair. The man had conspired with his wife to shield both children from this truth. The son felt that his father had been weak for not leaving his marriage after he realized that his wife was cheating. Of course, by the end of the one-hour program (things are so easily resolved on TV), the son sees that his father was actually a man of tremendous strength who chose to forgive his wife and raise her child as his own in order to keep his family together.

My own father closed his eyes to my mother's extramarital affair, too. Perhaps it was not out of weakness, as I had also always believed. Perhaps he kept silent to save his family. My dad hoped that my mother's affair would run its course. In a weird way, that TV show helped me recognize my father's strength. Of course, our personal situation was more complex than that presented in the TV show. As much as my father's God and his religion helped him endure through the lean times, he lacked the tools necessary to speak an emotional/spiritual language that we children needed in the midst of a very confusing situation. We needed an anchor and a guide-wire, but my father was not adept. My mother's heart was closed to the repercussions her affair had upon us children, as well. Keeping us at bay allowed her to evade the consequences of her choices. She was not forced to reckon with her actions. And we all flounder in the fallout, still.

Jane and I vacationed in Tucson. We drove to an outcropping of pictographs drawn centuries ago by the Hohakum Indians. I sat on the ground near a grouping of sandstone rocks and listened to the wind. My heart urged me to know that my speaking voice will come back in full force. I needed to be patient. I am being prepared for something that will be revealed when the timing is right.

The next day, we drove to Phoenix and visited the Heard Museum. I was drawn to a display of Pueblo battle shields. Constructed of animal hides, then painted and decorated, they hardly seemed as if they would protect the bearer, they were so small. Each shield contained a spiritual emblem that felt more powerful than metal or armor. Stability, cohesion, and wholeness were embodied in each shield; each possessed a directness and a simplicity that was at once sparse and ornate.

What struck me most was that none of the shield designs was psychologically fragmented. None of the images was confusing or disjointed like a Picasso or a Salvador Dali painting. Absent was the sense of alienation. The human spirit emanating from each shield was not broken. The power of communication and connection, of utility and cultural expression, of community and lineage was everywhere evident.

Recovery is excruciating. To accept where I am right now and bathe it in loving-kindness is not an abstract concept. It is quite real, very concrete. And extremely difficult. It hits me where I live. It's a simple concept, but enacting it is painstaking.

I talked with Beth about needing to slow down, have fun, and take care of myself in tender ways. She suggested that I do small things, like taking a hot bath, looking at ice crystals on the windowpane, dunking molasses cookies into hot tea, playing music, letting myself know that life is full of mystery, wonder, beauty.

The paper-white bulbs that Jane and I forced are arching their long, green-fingered stems toward the window, seeking sunshine. What is alive is insistent, even through the cold and the dark. Light reaches for life.

It dipped to -33 degrees last night just shy of the 1970 record of -34 degrees. The high today is -10! The weatherman on WCCO invited viewers to visit the North Star Ice Company if they wanted to escape the cold. He said it was a balmy 18 degrees above zero inside the warehouse! A full 31 degrees warmer than it was at the moment of his forecast (-13 degrees below). I laughed out loud at the absurdity of it all. Visiting an ice warehouse suddenly held tropical appeal. Yesterday, I boiled water and then tossed it outside. The hot liquid vaporized as it hit the frigid air. It was startling to witness that physical manifestation of the cold. This winter is just too brutal.

Sales of *No Matter What* are plummeting. No marketing campaign to sustain book sales and a writer who can't read her work out loud to help promote it. Sorry state of affairs. I need to trust that the book will get the exposure it deserves—eventually. People will buy it, read it, and perhaps through word of mouth, sales will improve until I am able to lend it my full support again. Low book sales is not a punishment for my inability to do readings nor is it a punishment for my having broken the silence of family secrets.

I read a whole chapter of my sequel-in-progress out loud at my writers group this week. I didn't make it through the chapter perfectly, but I kept reading, kept trying. There were times when I ran out of air, times when I felt choked. There were also times when my voice was clear and loud and the words flowed smoothly. When I finished, the women said, "Yeah! You did it!"

As a kid, when I was experiencing the traumas of abuse, my psyche/spirit/mind left, but my body had no similar escape route. My body recorded the truth of my experiences even as everything and everyone around me minimized or denied my reality. What I realized in therapy this week was that my body is the Witness Bearer, the ultimate Truth Teller. *It holds tight so I won't minimize or forget.* If I fail to honor my past and its repercussions, my body will hold harder to its truth.

Instead of trying to disassociate and be a person who thinks her abuse was in the past and was really *not so bad,* I must name the damage. I am a survivor. I need to lay down my burdens as well as those many bundles that do not belong to me—the grief and anger and fear that belong to my mother, my siblings, and my father. I must return their wounds and deal with my own, which are plentiful enough.

Through Hakomi, I am trying to learn how to empower my body to express in deeper and more profound ways. I can give my body the tools it needs to respond with less clenching. Beth said that this will be a lifelong process, but eventually, the re-patterning will be accomplished. The parts of me that hold the consciousness of my trauma can evolve to a place where they don't control my entire body. The default urge to tense will always be with me, but it won't be the only response from which I can choose.

A few days ago, I felt a subtle shift in my breathing. My belly opened and eased. My breath rose from a deeper place in my body. The foundation was more solid, more spacious. I breathed, fully, for the first time in a very long time.

I haven't been sleeping well. This sadness is older than my present struggle between my ego and my body. It lives in the memory of what my body has endured, the grief it has collected and stored. Change is incremental. No big release. No lightning bolts. No geological shifts. Just the slow accumulation of new ways. It takes so much *damned* time.

I am starting to feel sadness *in* my body. My numbness is thawing.

The thawing loosens other feelings, especially anger. My tense speech barks at my face. I can't control it. I never know when I try to speak if my voice is going to sound strained or easy.

I need a reprieve from the stress of it. Will my voice work this time? Will I be able to communicate verbally what I am feeling? Thinking? What I believe? Speech is something most people take for granted. I don't any longer. I am angry. I am unable to trust that my body will support me in my efforts to function on an everyday level. It's as if I have a disability without the explanation for it. Or the understanding from others. If I were confined to a wheelchair, no one would expect me to get up and walk, but nobody has any idea of the impairment of my voice until I begin to speak.

It feels as if my parasympathetic synapses are running amok. How do I point to those things in the context of my daily life? How do I explain that there is a reason for this? I am having a severe reaction to childhood trauma. Some people's bodies "cope" by getting cancer. My body "copes" by strangling my speech. It's getting tougher to handle.

I've been finding comfort in reading Pema Chödrön and listening to her tapes about maitri, loving-kindness. Pema says that before one can attain the advanced stage of loving-kindness, she must be able to do maitri for herself. Unless this is accomplished, compassion toward others is less than authentic. However, this practice is not about being good or doing it right. It's about planting the seeds of maitri and trusting that they will germinate and grow at their own rate. The opportunity is to see that there is no difference between one's self and one's enemies. And there is no difference between what one would call one's personal demons and the aspects of one's personality that one freely embraces and labels as good. Every human being longs for happiness and love and an end to the suffering of life. We are the same at the most essential level. And that core is loving-kindness.

While this Tonglen practice is fundamental and simple, it is very difficult. Most Westerners find it daunting to bathe themselves in self-love and self-acceptance. It is too painful, and by cultural standards it is also considered selfish, but maitri practice is not about Ego. It's not about acquiring; it's about opening to what arises. The energy is necessarily different. And so is the outcome.

114

Chapter 16

I want my voice back, goddamnit!! I'm pissed. I want to scream and shout and yell, "I'm mad! I'm mad! I want my voice back!!!!!"

I am depressed and despairing. Sleeping is increasingly difficult. I feel overwhelmed with angst about my voice. Hakomi and psychotherapy take so much energy. I want to collapse into a deep sleep and not wake until my body figures out how to do this differently. I've been thinking about going to see an acupuncturist for support of my body's parasympathetic nervous system. Part of me holds back, trying to ascertain if this course of action is coming from my head, from my need to "fix it."

I *do* want to fix my voice. I want to be able to speak again without strain or tension. If I could figure out how to get my voice back, reliably, I'd do it. I'd still do my therapy and my Hakomi work, but I think I would feel less stress in my life if I could just *talk*. It would be such a huge relief. Is it physical? Is speech therapy the answer?

Panic. Panic. Panic. Fear. Grief. Anger. My gut aches with them all. My breathing shallows. My temples pound. My head aches. There is no exit, no way for these hostile feelings to emerge. I imagine a volcano spewing lava, smoke and ash into the air, hot and riled. My emotions are high. My voice is tense. I am ovulating. The tightness waits for my blood to flow. My neck muscles harden. The words are trapped in my throat.

How long can I endure this?

My life is changing, drastically, in deep emotional ways, but progress is painstaking. During a therapy session I broke down and asked Anne to help me over this hurdle of frustration and impatience. She said she would. She told me she had witnessed much growth and healing in me. She said that I more easily allow myself to have feelings and to name them. I cry more readily, now, instead of holding back. I confront shame when it arises. She encouraged me to continue to use my painting and my clay to externalize what my body is feeling. In this way, I can give my body support and show it that it no longer has to keep secrets to feel safe. She suggested that I look at my art pieces as a monument to my survival.

Later that week, Beth suggested that we blow bubbles as part of our Hakomi session. I said, "In the house?" and laughed at myself for sounding so parental. Beth and I blew bubbles, listening to classical music. At first, I felt dumb and far removed from the grown-up I was supposed to be. Eventually, I relaxed and had fun.

Everyone is intent on helping me. I mentioned to my youngest sister, Peg, who is a psychiatric medical resident, that I had been having a couple of hard weeks. She asked me whether I would consider taking anti-depressants. I told her I didn't feel I was debilitated most of the time. What was really frustrating me was my voice. She replied, "I hate to say this, but since you feel it's related to panic and anxiety, meds would probably help with your voice, too."

It's tough to say no to anti-depressants when I am feeling as if I am at the end of my rope. The alternative healing choices I have made are slower to show progress. A deeper, more organic healing takes longer. I get impatient. The lure of a drug that might make me less anxious so that my voice would return is quite seductive.

I discussed my sister's suggestion with Jane. She wants more information about the side-effects of anti-depressants. She doesn't want to see me jump at a magic bullet fix. I am torn. Maybe the drugs could help. I am going to try an alternative, first. I learned about a Chinese herbal formula that is supposed to combat anxiety. I'll use it for a month and see if it helps. I'll also talk to Anne about anti-depressants and see what information she has and ask her opinion.

This week, I cried about being taken from my brothers and my father. I didn't focus on the details; I just felt the raw restlessness of the emotion—for the first time, ever.

The time is drawing near to let grief go. After all these years, I am safe now. I am strong enough. Holding on made sense before. I had no place to put it. Now I do. I can leave it on the floor in Anne's office. I can give it to the wind. I can let the waters of Lake Superior wash it away. I can release it without discounting the trauma or the loss of my childhood. I no longer need it to survive. I no longer have to live in an unsafe house terrorized by my mother's emotional instability, my brothers' angst, my own jailed rage. I no longer have to grieve my father's emotional absence. He escaped. How did he do that?

Why didn't he take me with him?

It is time to open my ribs and let it all pour out. I give my body permission to *feel* the grief instead of *be* grief.

I showed my drawings of grief masks and voice masks to Anne. Afterward, I wanted to crawl into a fetal curl and cry, *I hurt. I hurt.* Over and over, I coaxed myself to soften and open. I told myself that my *aversion* to the pain was the real culprit. That is what made me tense. I also tried to be less critical of my need to hold on, if that is what felt safest.

Later, at home, I shoveled the walks and then went inside and pushed against the door jamb, breathing through the exertion. I screamed. Afterward, I drew two pictures of hands pushing things away.

On International Women's Day, my mother called to make a breakfast date. It has been a long time since we have seen each other. I think I am ready. After the phone call, I had a fantasy about having a heart-to-heart chat with her. In that fabricated conversation, I said that instead of fearing death and all Mom feels she has to pay back to her Maker, she might consider working it out with her kids. Atonement and self-forgiveness. We both need that. We both need to forgive one another.

Yesterday, my diaphragm was tight, even with the Chinese anti-anxiety supplements. Instead of fighting it, I said, "Okay, voice. Come on in. Stay as long as you need to. You are welcome here." I meant it. I'm tired of fighting. My tense voice is not a reflection of my worth as a human being. I just have a tight diaphragm. It's the way my body holds its tension. End of discussion. Some days I wake up and my shoulder is sore. I don't jump to conclusions. I don't tell myself that I am a defective person because my shoulder aches. Why should I make that leap when it is my diaphragm that is tight? Or my speech?

Trusting my process without shaming or judging is very difficult. I am asking myself to re-arrange the old, mircd patterns and replace them with something kinder, less harmful. I have to learn to disengage from the outcome. Whether I get my voice back or not.

I have been having curious dreams. Subconscious movies.

I dreamt I had been invited to my college reunion, but I didn't want to attend. I didn't want to be closeted returning to a gathering at that Catholic women's college. On the day of the reunion, I drove to the campus to spy on the happenings. I watched a group of women preparing for the opening procession of alumnae and teachers. A woman added my name to the list of those they had been unable to contact. I felt sad. Part of me wanted to participate in the reunion, see old college friends, but I didn't want to pretend to be straight. I didn't want to be silent about my real life. I felt that I had to choose between personal integrity and my connection with the college.

My absence at the reunion felt like a price that I had to pay to protect myself. I cried as I watched the academic procession. My tears surprised me. Back at the front gate, several women recognized me. "Why aren't you coming to the reunion?" they asked. Then a woman who had been in my graduating class walked to the gate and sat in another woman's lap. They were very affectionate. The woman introduced my ex-classmate to me before I could tell her that we already knew one another. My ex-classmate replied, "I don't know anything about your life. There's nothing written down about you." I stated,

"There's plenty written about my life. And I've written it."

This week Jane told me she had noticed my voice has improved over the past month. She thinks it's because I've been saying "no" more often and displaying more confidence.

For some strange reason, her comments made me think about the time I was eighteen and tried to stab myself in the diaphragm with a kitchen knife. I was distraught over my mother's disapproval of my coming out as a lesbian. Looking back, it is significant that I aimed the weapon at my diaphragm—the "shadow bag" as the author of the book *Guilt is the Teacher, Love is the Lesson* calls the shadow side. Inside this shriveled, tight bag I have stowed away my courage, my power, and my hard feelings. They are painful, and I am afraid. The irony is that they only immobilize me if I do not open the "bag" and shake out the contents.

I wish I could move this heaviness. I thought screaming might help, but I let out a wail, and it failed to satisfy me. I need tears, but the tears aren't forthcoming.

I had breakfast with my mother at a local restaurant. I tried to keep our conversation at the coffee-and-toast level, not let it dip into the more dangerous waters of emotions. I have so much I need to say to her, yet she is one of the hardest people for me to talk to. The waters are too treacherous. We can talk about gardening and cooking, my siblings or the weather but not the dangerous truths. I have to remember to float at the surface. I do miss her, but I can't visit her with the expectation that our relationship is the kind of mother-daughter bond that either one of us desires.

I try to recognize my mother's finer points. She has a wonderful sense of humor. She's a great cook. She can be very playful —girlish almost. And she loves to garden. At breakfast, Mom told me she was proud of who I grew up to be. She said she likes what she sees when she looks at me. When she added that she likes to think she played a part (even if a small part) in me ending up so well, my ambivalence surged. She did influence me, for good and for bad. She was my primary parent, but I have also done a great job of raising myself. I guess we have to share in the billing for the woman I have become.

Mom asked if I was writing. I said, "Yes. Remember I told you that I was working on a sequel to *No Matter What*." She responded, "You did?" "Yes," I replied. "Remember you said 'Who'd be interested in something like that?'"

She asked, "Am I gonna be able to read this one?" My mother has not been able to get past the fourth chapter of *No Matter What*. I replied, "I can't know that, Mom."

She emphasized how the first novel was too painful to read. It brought her back to a time in her life that was too hard to revisit. She said it was okay for me to write it and that she hoped it helped me heal. I tried to stay glassy-eyed, but my heart raged. She didn't acknowledge her need for healing, didn't own responsibility for her pain. She pushes it back onto me, making me the "sick" one who needs to heal, the one who is damaged. She didn't acknowledge that she, too, is bruised. Her wounds led her to choices that had dire consequences for herself and for her children.

Maybe someday, we will be able to talk with honesty and clarity about our messy legacy. For now, that time will have to wait.

Jane and I saw the movie *Antonia's Line*. The film's main character, Antonia is a self-assured woman who is a wise, compassionate warrior. (My dream mother!) Antonia is no goody-goody, though. She has her rage and her faults, but she creates a loving environment in which her daughter and granddaughter—and an assortment of village castaways—gather round. This collection of people flourish in Antonia's presence because, instead of controlling others, she allows room for everyone to be fully who they are.

In one scene, Antonia confronts the town bully after he has raped her granddaughter in an act of revenge against Antonia's daughter. Antonia stands before the rapist, gun in hand, but she doesn't kill him. Instead, she curses him. She calls down the powers of heaven to do her bidding. She banishes him from the community, telling him that if he ever dares return, everything he touches will sour. That scene was immensely powerful. Antonia did not accept or acquiesce to his abuse. She was fiercely protected by her own integrity.

I brought this deep wish for a mother like Antonia into my therapy session this week. I sobbed hard. Snot ran from my nose; tears poured. I told Anne about my breakfast with my mother and the headache that I had after I went home. I told her how my mother had said, "Breakfast was nice. Let's not wait two years to do that again."

I talked about the pain I felt hearing my mother's comments about my writing. That is a place where the shame grabs hold tightly. No matter how hard I try, I still believe that in writing *No Matter What,* I tattled on my mother. I told the whole world that things weren't as great as we pretended they were. I felt angry and patronized by my mother's remarks about how, if writing that novel helped me heal, it was okay with her. I told Anne that if I could, I would say to my mother, "I wish you'd own your part in this whole ordeal."

Anne replied, "Say it, then. Say it here, right now, with me."

I tried, but I couldn't muster the courage. Saying it once took every ounce of fortitude I had.

Defying my mother is too risky. A comment such as, "I wish you'd own your part in this whole ordeal," might not seem so menacing on the surface, but it is really a usurpation of her power in my family. It smacks of disloyalty. It reeks of selfishness and cruelty when viewed through the lens of the familial rule: *love Mother at all costs*.

I sobbed for not being able to assert my truth, not even to an invisible mother in a room far across town, safe in the presence of my therapist. A deeper understanding emerged. My primary feeling toward my mother was neither love nor anger, but fear.

I shook as I admitted, out loud, "I do not love my mother." I sobbed—heavy, remorseful sobs—as if my tears could redeem me from this most grievous of all sins.

Anne sat next to me then. She affirmed, "You don't owe your mother love. Love and trust and respect are things one earns."

I told her that I worried the Mommy Police were going to throw me in jail. She told me to tell them that my therapist said I didn't have to go. She also said, "You'll still go to Heaven even if you don't love your mother, Mary. You don't need to have the compassion of the Dalai Llama or of Mother Teresa."

I am a lost, aching hole of sadness and loneliness. I feel responsible, yet not at all responsible. This messy stew of emotions is relentless. I am mad that my mother let me down, that it has always been such hard work, always take-take-take. I have waited a long time to tell my truth, and now telling it scares me. This secret has transformed itself into blood and bones and skin. I cannot extricate myself from it. To do so would be to disown my own body. If I let the secret out, will my bones splinter? Will they puncture my skin? Bleed blood upon the floor until I breathe no longer?

I have spent my life keeping my deepest Self from my mother, afraid that she would take that from me as well. In doing so, I have kept the world from my deepest Self. Some part of me agreed to expose my heart through my writings. Maybe there is a deepest Self within the deeper Self, something more eternal, more enduring than the story-line of my particular saga, something that is grounded in Truth, something that feels safe and calm, anchored to a bigger more spacious heart. As a child, silence equaled life and protection, pseudo-safety in a terrifyingly unreliable world. More and more I realize that speaking the truth equals life.

I want to live, not die.

I want to live.

I dreamt that someone intent on killing me was assaulting me. There was blood everywhere. In another dream, a burglar was trying to rob my house but I caught him in the act and he left. I took off and fell in with a crowd that was trying to control me. I kept trying to speak my own truths, name my own reality, and challenge the others. One man in particular was trying to control what others said, wore, and did. I kept ranting, "No, that's not how I see it! No! I don't believe that at all!"

Chapter 17

I feel antsy, irritable. I've been editing my sequel, *Finding Grace*. The work itself stirs up old losses. I need to meditate, then scream or dance to move the rough energy. The story is about an un-mothered child who tries to grow up fast and take care of her younger sister. The old ghosts poke at me, reminding me of my own mother-grief. Can I release these apparitions? Send them off to their final resting-place?

My days have been dark and dreary; hope is elusive. I day-dream about being admitted to a psych ward, thinking it would somehow allow me to step out of my life and dance this torrid tango in a contained environment, away from the day-to-day demands of my life. My Chinese anti-anxiety pills are dwindling. I'm down to twelve tablets and I have been rationing them, lowering the dosage and skipping the number of times I am supposed to take them in an attempt to stretch out the remaining pills. Maybe that's part of why I feel so jittery. They are my herbal Prozac.

The shame I feel around my tense voice has been biting. It takes a lot of energy to prep myself before I call a business colleague, a client, or a friend on the phone. I psyche myself like a reluctant athlete. "You can do it," I urge. "You are strong." I call on my archetypes, Crone, the mother-protector and Warrior, the woman of courage. I ask God and my Spirit Guides for support. I jump up and down and scream to release the fear trapped in my diaphragm. After the phone calls, my body shakes, and I scream again trying to exorcise the tension. I can't stand it. It's tearing me up inside.

I'm still thrashing about with these terrible voice struggles. I am still staring in the mirror at the scared six-year-old version of myself. How long must this go on?

Thinking it would help calm my anxiousness, I went for a walk to the Lake Harriet band shelter, but my stewing was so distracting that I hardly noticed the swollen buds on the trees, the crows cawing in the branches, the ice still on the lake. The wind was chilly, but I endured the walk. I wanted it to be spring so badly. This winter has been demanding and exhausting, physically, emotionally, spiritually, and psychically. The Winter of my Discontent. Ha-ha. I'd laugh if I had the strength. So much withered skin to shed.

This strangled voice of mine is intimately entwined with my sense of authenticity. Being unable to grab what I want in the world is how my childhood traumas are most pointedly played

126

out in my adult life. An ancient part of my psyche believes I do not have a right to exist. *No Matter What* shoved my nose into this lie. My novel is a gift that has nudged me to unfetter the truth hiding inside the falsehood. I yearn to know what my life could be.

I dreamt I was in Tuscany with my sisters and my father. We were joined by a group of children and a rigid, controlling older woman. We were supposed to attend a funeral. The harsh woman told me to be quiet. This upset me, and I cried and sought comfort from my sisters. I was angry that my grief was not honored. The parental figures in the dream never wanted me to experience it in their presence. I took a walk to get out of the house and breathe.

The astrologer I saw in 1994 told me that these past few years were about getting myself spiritually sturdy. To accomplish this I must *feel* my anger and fear and grief. I understand that now. Crone is *me*. Warrior is *me*. Artist is *me*. Truth-Teller is *me*. Each is part of the singular whole—a splendid inner-mother who can cherish me.

More and more, I am preparing to grapple with my anger. Slowly, I am beginning to believe that my strained voice is *not* the result of being defective. It is the result of my body not being ready. That's a *huge* difference. I have no antidote for defectiveness. Preparation I can influence.

My creative work lives in my body as much as it lives in my mind, my heart, and my soul. With each painting, each clay sculpture, each manuscript, I reclaim pieces of my Self. I learn to listen to the wisdom of my body, when it resists and when it doesn't, and honor what it remembers.

I need to move my body. Rake the leaves. Pick up sticks. Shove yard waste into plastic bags. Trim tree branches. Clear away old plant stems. I want to welcome all the plants that made it through this hellish winter. So long the wait. So cold and dark and quiet. Now, the green emerges, everywhere. Pockets of tulips, crocus, white snowdrops, and daffodil tips poke through the dark soil, clawing at the light. The rhododendron bushes already bear buds. The azaleas, too. The asters have sprung small green leaves. The sweet woodruff unfurls, as does the pachysandra. Our garden is a glorious explosion of mystery, power, spirit, and comfort. All in my own back yard.

I dreamt that I worked as a fry cook. During my shift, I eyed a piece of cake in the restaurant walk-in refrigerator. Later, at home, I told my friend Carol that I wanted to go back and eat that slice. The dream shifted, and I took the form of a man. Carol and I were driving back to the restaurant, but we weren't getting there fast enough to suit me. My impatience was growing. I pulled out an arsenal of weapons and began to do battle with the forces that were keeping me from that piece of cake. A bloody battle ensued. At one point, a bomb destroyed the restaurant, and a baby was injured. She was blown in half. She had no body parts below her ribcage. The baby had lost her diaphragm, her sex organs, and her legs. She was a bloody mess of chest, heart, head, and arms. Remarkably, she was still alive. The dream shifted again, and I became the baby's mother. I was on the TV news telling the world that my baby had been injured and that she would get better. I would love her and take good care of her.

Even when my mind feigns amnesia, my body possesses perfect recall. I cried and shivered through my therapy session this week. Anne asked me if the emotions I was experiencing were old or current. "Old stuff," I said. She asked me to open my eyes and focus on objects in the room, so I wouldn't re-traumatize myself. That helped, but still I cried. My body released its fear. "I'm scared," I sobbed.

After our session, I drove to Lake Harriet. I stared at the water. I thought about diving in and not coming up, sinking into oblivion. I decided that such a silly idea was just my Ego trying to save face. I went home, lay down, and calmed myself by imagining Crone holding me in her arms, rocking me, telling me, *It's okay. You're gonna be okay.*

Today, I read an article in *Orion* about a man who was traveling across the United States. On one of his stopovers at an RV camp in a county park, he met a family and befriended a young girl of seven or eight. The child followed this man everywhere, asking wonderfully curious questions. They were fellow seekers, aficionados of the natural world, watchers of detail and natural phenomena. They noticed small things that others missed—pennies abandoned on tracks, flattened by trains—and other objects of wonder and importance.

The girl adopted this man. She and her family had been at the campground for nearly three weeks because her father had gotten a job at a local factory. The girl was savvy; she knew the land and its secret treasures. She became the man's tour guide. She trusted him, and much to my delight, he didn't misplace or abuse that trust. As my eyes moved from sentence to sentence, I worried that he might hurt her in some way, but it never came to be.

That sacred bond preserved, even honored, brought to each of them a kind of friendship, a shared vision of the world with all of its excitement. The pair was able to connect, even though they were years apart in age and barely knew one another. Even when the girl pestered the man, urging him to come out of his tent and talk with her, there was a sense of endearment in her nagging and in his response. He pulled on his jeans and joined her—a simple gesture, a heartfelt reaction to how important the connection with her had become to him. He could have dismissed her as bratty and intrusive. Instead, he invited her into his life, for that brief time. I am confident that they were both enriched by their friendship.

Jane and I saw *For Our Daughters* at the Illusion Theater. This play/performance piece is about breast cancer and the importance of community/friendship/support in the healing process. The women featured in the video talked about how the love and caring of their friends and their families was critical to their treatment. Healing goes deeper than chemotherapy and operations. Removing the cancerous growths is but one step. People, too, are a sort of balm, a medicine that is powerful and redemptive. I know this has been true for me in my life as well.

My first therapist, Rosemary—the one I worked with before I met Anne—had an abiding spiritual influence on me. She nurtured me, guided me, cared about me. She was the first adult authority figure I fully trusted. I can't have a friendship with her. It's against the therapy rules, but Rosemary is the kind of woman I'd choose as my mother if I could go to the Mom Store at the mall and pick one out. Maybe wanting this external manifestation of mothering is foolish. I should learn to nurture and mother myself. I *am* doing that, or at least I'm trying. But it's not enough. I still want a real *live* person, a human mother.

My throat is a jail of tight muscles. My voice is locked inside. This day of all days. My sisters and their families are coming to Jane's and my house for Mom's seventieth-birthday surprise party. I am anxious, pacing the floor, waiting for their arrival. Maybe I am hosting this party as a way to prove to myself (and to Mom?) that I am a good daughter.

I am ambivalent about this gathering. I feel such deep anger at my mother. I can't have a relationship with her until I learn to let go. She isn't the mom I want, but she is the mother I have. Wishing won't alter that. The changes must come from accepting the reality of what I have and making room for it with as much compassion as I can muster. I will try to leave the self-criticisms and the mother-judgments in the backyard during Mom's party. I will try to keep my heart open and soft. If I cannot succeed in doing this, I hope I can have compassion for the resistance, the non-opening, the protection. I never know what's going to show up.

My mother was moved to tears by her birthday party. She kept saying "Nothing this good has ever happened to me. No one has ever done anything this nice for me. It's the best thing that has ever happened in my life."

After dinner, our friend Diane and her friend Martin arrived to play the accordion and the violin for us. Mom was surprised and thrilled all over again. Part of me felt truly generous. I felt good about cooking for my mother and arranging the concert, but ultimately, the generosity I was able to muster was polluted by a festering pool of abandonment. I wish I could have given the food and the music out of a deeper heart connection, a truer bond of gratitude to my mother for all her years of love and nurturing. My authentic emotion was the lack of trust I feel toward my mother's love for me. I managed to make it through the celebration because I was resolved to honor a woman who was turning seventy. I value such demarcations in people's lives—for my mother, a co-worker, a neighbor, or a complete stranger.

I dreamt that I raged at my mother and my stepfather. I told them I was pissed and that I was leaving—moving out of their house. I shouted and screamed, ranting at them.

This week, for the first time in my recollection, I shouted out loud, "I'm so mad at you, Mom!"

There was no delay between my anger and the expression of it. I sobbed and shouted as I scrubbed the pots and pans. Snot dripped down my nose as I yelled again, "I'm so mad at you, Mom!" I rushed for some Kleenex, wiping my sudsy hands on my pants. I stared at my red face, my puffy eyes, and seethed at the bathroom mirror, "You're seventy years old, for Christ's sake. How much longer are you gonna be around? Isn't it time to take care of business?"

I dreamt that I was pregnant. My swollen belly was hidden beneath my shirt so people couldn't tell by looking at me that I was expecting a child. I felt the physical sensations of carrying a child inside my enlarged belly. The muscles in my lower back were tight. I was excited about being pregnant, but I had worried Jane wouldn't be because she had been unsure as to whether she wanted us to have children. When I told her I was carrying our child, she kissed me.

I had an extremely bad bout with anxiety yesterday, which led to a constricted voice. The muscles in my neck throbbed by the end of the day. My throat ached. I flailed around in a sea of neurosis as my voice pinched and my anxiety rose, and I internally tried to talk myself to a calmer place. "You can do it, Mary," I coaxed. "You're good at this. You're safe." The only thing I didn't try to tell my fearful Self in the midst of one of these funks was, "I love you."

Chapter 18

I have finally arrived in the country called Anger. I am long overdue. It's as uncomfortable as hell. I am having a very difficult time talking. My voice is tense. I feel restless, ready to explode. I fear I can't contain what's inside. I worry that I am going to burst. I don't know how to let my anger emerge gracefully, so I stuff it to avoid making a mess or becoming totally overwhelmed. The pressure builds, and I feel hot and tight. At least this time, I am aware of how angry I truly am.

It is my own power I am restraining. If I can do this piece, I will have access to a larger reservoir of my own personal energy. I will feel more whole. This anger isn't rational. It doesn't make any sense in terms of who my mother and stepfather are to me now. Today, they are harmless people who love me. My rage is young and appropriate to deeds once done.

My mother's and stepfather's past actions harmed me, whether it was their intention or not. I truly believe it was not their intention, which has always made it subtly harder for me to validate my anger. They are not evil. They are merely wounded. I can understand that *and* still be pissed as hell.

To help me direct and release some of this anger, Anne and I did an exercise this week. I pushed back against Anne's outstretched hands until my rage was spent. Afterwards, I sighed, "At last." I felt a strange, unfamiliar, and awkward sensation of peace. The tense war had lessened. The cease-fire had begun. After untold years of hiding from gunfire, fighter-bombers, the roar of artillery, and the howl of screaming wounded, I heard silence and stillness. And surrender.

Beneath the pain and the loss of my particular familial story line lies one unflinching truth: my mother didn't share her heart with me. She deposited her pain. She told me she loved me every day of my life, trying to pass that off as motherly love. I feel ripped off. It could have been different between us. It could have worked. She reneged on her role as Mother.

The gig is up.

Slow down. Breathe. Breathe. Breathe. I am so anxious. Over what? Things churning in me about Mom. I am scared to do this piece. I know it's time. I know it's necessary. I know it's messy and unpredictable, and I haven't even plunged to the depths of it yet. I'm afraid of losing her. Of losing my identity as a daughter. I have a sense of the power of this process, the cost of it to me. I'm changing and that feels good as well as frightening. I bumble about like a hobo of the heart, tattered and gangly.

I am exhausted. Deeply tired. My cells crave respite. My heart craves tenderness. My body longs for a cease-fire, yearns to be done with it all.

To help ease the logjam of emotions, I danced to Gabrielle Roth's videotape "The Wave." I swayed and jumped, twirled and rocked. Afterward, my belly and diaphragm had softened. My breathing was neither deep nor shallow. It slowed to a peaceful rhythm. I was able to talk on the phone with ease. My voice held no tension. The breath beautifully supported my speech.

I read a chapter in Pema Chödrön's book *The Wisdom of No Escape*, in which she discusses how humans try to avoid inconveniences. Sometimes, we go out of our way to make life easy, soft, safe. Pema suggests that life is juiciest when it is inconvenient. A lot of good dharma work can be done in this non-safe zone. She wrote that how you react to inconvenience or interact with it shows you much about yourself. Do you engage it? Shun it? Are you able to let inconvenience just be an experience that flows through you?

Most of the time, I am thoroughly attached to my need for convenience. I am so easily irritated when things go awry. Sometimes, I try to let it be, but most times I cannot even do this. My very human self gets stuck in the petty parts, and I am not selfless and giving. I am pissed and upset, wanting *my way*. This is an invitation to learn more about my limitations, my safety needs, and my irritability. It's also an invitation to practice loving-kindness with whatever is present—attachment or non-attachment, irritability or surrender.

I am *livid*. Utterly full of rage that I still don't have my voice. It's been almost three years. That's a long time to wince every time I open my mouth to speak.

I'm mad at the whole goddamn world. I've got a bad attitude, and I don't give a rip. I'm mad as hell at my body for shutting down to such an extreme length. I'm mad at people who comment about my voice, making me feel even more selfconscious and shameful. I'm mad that I can't rely on speech to communicate. I'm pissed as hell at people who can simply open their mouths and talk without anxiety or shame.

I want my voice back. It belongs to me. I want it *now*! I want my throat to loosen, my diaphragm to soften, my breath to flow, my voice to sing out!

I dreamt that Nate died. I went to his funeral. I wanted to tell people about the sexual abuse, explain to them how my tears were not about sorrow for his death, but for what he did to me, what he had taken from me. I lost my sense of safety, my sense of trust in myself and in my body's ability to defend itself. I lost my childhood and a sense of belonging in the world. I lost the possibility of happiness for a very long time.

I sobbed during my Hakomi session this week. I cried, partly because of Beth's tender compassion and partly because of my own growing ability to finally let her kindness in. I am starting to believe that I deserve to take up more space in the world. Just enough so that I don't shrink away, entirely. Just enough to fill the edges of my own skin, comfortably.

What would my life be like without this harboring of sadness? I'd have more room for joy. I could feel the sorrow but not have to hold on to it. My feelings could rise and fall, come and go in their own natural rhythm. My muscles wouldn't have to clench and tighten.

I can't engage in a simple conversation with a close friend

without feeling the urge to crawl out of my skin. I have to stand up, pace the floor. I turn and twist my body in all manner of directions. Something wild, fierce, and fearful overtakes me. The stress mounts, and the panic consumes me. My throat clenches. My voice breaks. My heart sinks. Tears well up in my eyes.

Maybe I am coming to the proverbial Darkest Hour. Is all the work I've been doing bringing me to this place of deepest hurt, so I can push through to the other side? I try to pace it so I am not overwhelmed, but the anxiety has been constant these past three weeks. I woke at 5 a.m. stewing, ruminating about how extremely hard this all is. Every day takes every ounce of courage I can muster. Every day, I try to be brave and be present to what is. I lose faith so easily.

If my voice is still as huge an issue in six months, I'm going to consider anti-depressants. Maybe the body/mind connection for me also includes a chemical imbalance. Maybe it's more primal, more cellular than I can imagine or cope with. Maybe meds are just another form of support, among many.

My friend Karen talked about anger being a slow-moving lava flow. It destroys everything in its path. It purges. Anger is a cleansing, truly honest emotion. I need to let her words sink in. The outward thrust toward anger is colliding with the inward tensing of old constricting habits. Anger is the part of me that is newest, freshest, and most unsure. It is also rightfully, completely mine, totally genuine and ingenuous. To claim it is the hardest of tasks even though it is my greatest desire. I pray that I can keep moving, screaming, crying, letting the process run its course.

Can I learn to see anger as a gift—a blessing bestowed by Spirit to protect and uphold my soul and the integrity of my humanity? Anger that defines a limit, a boundary, anger that reclaims personal power and self-respect, anger over injustice and mistreatment—this is God-Anger. God expressing displeasure. Sacredness has been violated. I am a part of the Divine, and the Divine abides in me. Something Godly was violated through the abuses and traumas of my childhood. And I am mad as hell about it.

Chapter 19

Steven Spielberg is spearheading a nationwide/international effort to videotape interviews with Jewish survivors of the Holocaust. A Minneapolis freelance writer volunteered to interview people for the project. In a newspaper article, the writer talked about witnessing the stories and about the necessity of remembering. She said that as she listened to the horrors and evils of the brutality, she was moved to tears by how these women and men survived.

One Jewish woman recalled a Yiddish lullaby her mother—

who didn't survive the death camps—had sung to her when she was a child. I thought of the power of Spirit's will to live, of its ability to transcend human cruelty. It may survive wounded. It may be fragmented and scarred, but it survives. Spirit craves life.

How does one heal from such abject abuse and trauma? So many of these women and men never told their stories because they were cautioned, "Don't talk about it. The past is the past. Not in front of the children." All the many ways we learn to bury our suffering, distance ourselves from the unbearable pain. I think of the healing that comes with the telling, the power of naming one's experience. I think of how crucial that has been in healing from my own traumas, which pale in comparison to the atrocities of the Nazi death camps. I remember that while forgiveness is important in healing, so is remembering.

Always forgive but never forget. Forgetting is a form of self-abuse. Forgiving and remembering are intrinsic elements of self-love. The intent is not to dwell on the abuse, not to wallow in it, but rather to know and to claim your own personal history, to witness your life, with all its pain and joys. And to honor where you have been and where you have yet to go. Remembering allows you to come home to your own heart. How can a person truly be free if she doesn't acknowledge and embrace who she is at her roots? She would always be trying to run away, seeking solace from strangers, seeking refuge from something she can never outrun.

We carry our past in every cell. Consciousness is formed and sent into the world with every breath. Inhale. Exhale. Forgive. But never forget. I can't go forward unless, and until, I bring the past with me.

I dreamt that I was leaving home, again. My third such dream this week. In this one, I told my mother I had to go in order to do my writing. I told her writing was what I had come to the planet to do,

140

and I needed to honor this. My mother, and others, mocked me. "Oh, you think you're such a good writer. You ain't so hot. Who cares about what you write about? Who'd want to read it?" I got mad and told them I didn't care what they thought. I knew what I needed to do and nothing was going to stop me.

CBS *Sunday Morning* did a piece about Gerda Kline, the woman who wrote *Everything Except My Life,* a book about her experience as a teenager in the Nazi death camps. Kline is now an old woman who writes, tours, and talks to kids about not giving up. She emphasizes the sanctity of life and the goodness that is possible in humanity. She says that she is most troubled when she hears of a teenager committing suicide. She wants kids to know that *the darker the night, the brighter the dawn.* Nothing is more precious than life. She said that in all her years in the death camps she never saw kids kill themselves or have a nervous breakdown. Even in that most horrible of places, Gerda Kline felt hope. She said she lived for her liberation, not her death.

So, too, on a different level did another writer, Lucy Grealy, who wrote *Autobiography of a Face.* Grealy's book is an interesting account of a young girl whose face is disfigured as a result of countless reconstructive surgeries, which the author underwent during her childhood in the aftermath of cancer of the jawbone. I liked the book, but I kept wishing that Grealy had written more about the emotional connections between herself, her parents, and her twin sister. I wondered, especially, about her relationship with her twin. What it must have added to Grealy's own pain to grow up with a mirror image of what she could have looked like without the jaw cancer and the subsequent ordeal that it brought to her. Grealy's story, however, was subtly powerful—gritty and honest.

Her book touched a raw wound in me. It caused me to reflect upon my voice struggles and how difficult it is to be different in the world. It is hard to constantly confront people's ignorance and cruelty, harder still to face one's own selfconsciousness and shame.

I rarely talk about my father in my sessions with Anne. He is a mute ghost sitting in the chair across the room—as if I sprang solely from my mother's womb with no biological connection to him. Oh, how I wish I could have a relationship with at least one of my parents.

This week, I broke my subconsciously imposed father-silence. I cried as I told Anne how it felt to be taken from my father. I sobbed when I related his emotional distancing before my mother ran off with my sisters and me. Through snot and sniffles, I told Anne, "If I talk about Dad, I have to talk about getting in the car on that September afternoon in 1967 and leaving him. Not ever being able to say good-bye or tell him that I missed him."

I still bear enormous guilt and responsibility for my mother's decision to leave. What if I had said *no* when my mother asked me if we should go? Would that have changed everything? Would we have stayed? Would it have just delayed our departure, postponed it to another day? Why didn't I at least try to stop my mother from leaving? Anne reminded me that the decision to run away wasn't my responsibility. I was just ten days shy of my thirteenth birthday. She said my mother would have gone anyway, but I am not so sure.

If I had refused, maybe Mom would have read my desperation. I didn't fully understand the consequences of leaving—how irreversible it was. Part of me wanted to go. I wanted out of my own pain. I wanted to escape my parents' bickering and the taunts and teasing of my brothers. I wanted to be far, far away from Nate. I wanted to erase the English test I'd flunked that morning at school. I wanted to run hard and fast and long from the whispers and stares of townspeople gossiping about my mother's affair. I ached to be released from the myriad prisons that threatened to lock me out of a future of hope and happiness. Some part of me believed that my soon-to-be stepfather could ease the emotional burden of my mother, provide her with an adult to rely on, freeing me to be just a kid once more. As it turned out, I was wrong about that. He was envious of my relationship with my mom and turned his jealousy against me. And I didn't, couldn't realize, then, how much I would miss my father and my brothers. I hadn't counted on how deeply it would hurt to be away from them.

I can't retrieve the touch of my father's hand on my face the morning of the day we left—before I knew it would be the last time I would see him for two years. There is no machine, no pill, no gifted therapist that can make me thirteen again and transport me home to my father's house. All I can do now is give myself the gift I was refused nearly thirty years ago. All I can do is wail at the loss, honor the injustice, and curse the twist of fate that exiled me from him.

During my Hakomi session this week, I tried to be cognizant of the differences between my left and my right shoulders. My left felt airy, light, energized while my right felt tight, stiff, pained, stubborn. Beth asked if I could receive this information without judging it. Both shoulders possessed their own wisdom, she said. My left shoulder could teach my right shoulder how to release. My right shoulder could teach me the wisdom behind its holding on.

Non-dualism is a difficult concept for me to retain. The right side could be good in its refusal to open. I could love it as much, see it as valuable as the left side's ability to be calm and relaxed. How to hold the paradox, accept the sagacity of both?

I am still wrestling with guilt, trying to forgive myself for not saying no to my mother the day that she took my sisters and me away from Dad and our brothers. Anne asked me if I could offer myself even just a tiny token of forgiveness. I retraced the steps that led to our leaving that autumn afternoon, searching for some shard of absolution. I recalled how my mother and her boyfriend had told us girls that we were going to move, someday, and be a family. They said that we could choose our favorite place, either Magic City or Dream City—which were their names for Minneapolis and St. Paul, Minnesota, respectively. They promised that we could eat chocolate cake for supper there, if we wanted. We could sleep in canopied beds, and we'd each have a shiny, new bicycle to call our own.

I remembered believing them. The harsh reality of my life at home paled against this happy rendering of our soon-to-be family.

My life under my father's and mother's roof was far less glamorous.

My father was a machinist at the local pump factory. He supported seven kids and a wife on a workingman's salary. Too many bills and not enough paycheck strained his marriage to my mother and made him too weary to take an active role in the upbringing of his children. We had little except a roof over our heads. We never ate out. We were limited to one glass of milk every day. And we often wore hand-me-downs from older cousins.

On the few occasions that my mother did trot me downtown to the local clothing store for something new, I would cower behind racks of skirts and dresses as she brought our purchases to the cashier. The saleswomen knew that we could not afford the items, knew that our family had a mounting overdue bill that my father made earnest, if futile, attempts to pay off over time.

We were far from rich, by any standards—far from middle class as well. The finer luxuries of life were quite foreign to me— reserved for movie stars in fan magazines and celebrities on TV shows. The whimsical musings and fantastical promises that my mother and her boyfriend spun were literally the stuff of dreams, well beyond the realm of my small-town, working-class world. Why wouldn't I want all the wonderful things they vowed we would have after we moved?

The answer to Anne's question about forgiving myself arose with sudden clarity. "I could forgive myself for being naïve, for being duped and seduced by stories about magical, dream cities." I told her. "If I tried hard, I could forgive how impressionable I was."

"That's a start," Anne said.

Guilt is a shield that deflects my rage. I am angry with my mother for putting the onus of leaving on my non-quite thirteen-year-old shoulders. I had to say *yes* for her because she couldn't. She abdicated her responsibilities as the forty-one-year-old grownup, and I have carried that burden, ever since. Can I stay with that anger? Can it help purge the guilt that consumes me for having said *yes*? I don't know.

That September day in 1967 forever changed my life. Instead of stomping my feet, yelling *take me home!* out the car window, kicking my soon-to-be-stepfather in the shins, I stuffed my anger, shoved it deep into the pit of my belly. I couldn't afford to feel it back then. I twisted it into self-blame and hyper-responsibility. The Judas-price was my own safety. Mom would protect me, take me away with her, make me visible. I disowned my anger, lost my chance to voice my rage.

In the years afterward, as my new life unfolded in Minnesota, I couldn't afford to be a frivolous teenager. I couldn't waste precious time worrying about pimples and training bras. I had to solve my family's vast problems, choose between my mother and my father. Pretend that each Thanksgiving, each Christmas, every birthday party without Dad and my brothers was of no consequence. *I didn't need them*, I told myself countless times, *I have a new family now, a better family,* but I knew that was a lie, a falsehood that caught in my throat. Time and time again I swallowed the jagged truth of my anger, concealing it from my mother and from myself.

Forgiveness begins by absolving myself for wanting to survive, wanting more for myself, for hoping in the possibilities that leaving Seneca Falls offered, for trusting my mother, for believing that she and her boyfriend could make my life better. Maybe the silly dreams of my young heart weren't so silly after all. Maybe the time has come to spit out the lies and clear the anger from my throat before I choke to death.

This week, I attended the funeral of a colleague's mother. During the service, a man read a letter written to the deceased woman by one of her daughters. It talked of their warm and loving relationship. My heart tightened, thinking about how hard it will be for me when my mother dies—especially if she passes on before we fully reconcile. When my panic subsided, I realized that whatever happens, happens. I can't control when she or I will leave this life and fretting about that, now, is unproductive, wasteful. It keeps me trapped in the submissive role of the good girl who is too afraid to embrace anger, embrace the fact that the storybook mother-daughter relationship for which I long is a fantasy.

I didn't have it.

I won't have it.

Ever.

Chapter 20

Learning to grapple with my anger has been hard on my body. I don't always know how to release the knots of emotion. Shards of rage are stuck in cubbyholes of muscle, unable to find the pathway out. Anxiety is rampant. I've been seeing a chiropractor for treatment to relieve a pinched nerve in my left shoulder. She said the symptoms—or recognition of the problem via aches and pains—sometimes come quite a while after the body has actually been in distress. I have a subluxation, which the doctor's pamphlet said could be caused by physical, emotional, and mental stress. A riot of feelings is reverberating off my muscles and bones. My insides are torqued. I am hoping that the chiropractic care will prove to be a roadmap, providing my anger with a passageway through the labyrinth.

I did voice toning yesterday. Sitting in the sunlight on a pillow in our sunroom, I took a deep breath, relaxed, and opened my mouth. Powerful sounds arose. Growls and angry howls, sorrowful and wailing. Lilting, musical tones, too. The bones in my face vibrated. So did my ribs.

Sometimes, my voice caught. Sometimes it released, determined to stay open. Other times it faltered. Unable to maintain its clarity, it cracked. Tense and tired, it succumbed to my clenched throat muscles.

These bone-chilling sounds surprised me. It was good to hear the timbre of my own voice—with all its idiosyncrasies, its scratchiness, its power, its cadence, its joy, its sorrow, its rage. To hear myself *out loud*. Like a self-possessed diva, I belted out a *big voice*. Loud. Resounding. Amazing.

I went to my Hakomi session this week, weary of the constant pinched-nerve pain in my left side. As Beth worked on me, I concentrated on breathing deeply and eventually emotions surfaced. I sobbed harder and harder. Beth asked, "Are there words that go with those feelings?" I didn't respond, choosing not to usurp the rawness with intellectual analysis.

In letting the tears flow, without the circumvention of explanation, I allowed frustration and rage to rush from my wailing mouth. I knew *exactly* who I was angry at and why, but more important, I *felt* the anger and I let it fly. I reached under Beth's bodywork table and gripped the wooden supports to steady my body as I gave into the rampage of feelings. That anchor helped me ride the powerful buzzing in my veins.

What I was experiencing bore no resemblance to a rational,

sane discourse. This time, anger was a thing of bone and muscle, blood and breath. I was a body *feeling*, uncensored. Snot and tears and deep crying. Stomping feet and balled-up fists. I was *present* at this party. With *no* shame, no guilt.

Later, at home, I sat in the sunroom again and did another toning session. I opened my mouth and sound rushed from the core of my belly. I listened to my loudness and marveled, trying to visualize myself with a confident speaking voice. I possessed such an instrument, once. I catch glimpses of it every now and then. At those times, when my voice rings clear and strong, my heart quickens. *There she is,* I tell myself. *That's the voice I remember.*

I dream the possibility of my old voice returning, perhaps stronger for having endured this trial. If I can't believe it is possible, it won't happen. *Act as if* is an old Alcoholics Anonymous saying. Until a normal voice becomes a truer reality, until I can grow back into myself with power and grace and compassion, I can visualize it, will it into being.

I experienced long periods of great anxiety this week. I felt trapped and fearful about my voice for days on end. How do I get fierce enough to reclaim it? How do I get sturdier? Harder? More forceful? I need to get tough and stay tough, so that I don't fold into a wimpy clump of crumpled paper. Where did my confidence go? *And why?*

To loosen the grip of fear, I drew somber, dark, menacing images with oil pastels. Faces with open, crying mouths, sad tortured eyes. I fantasized about looking into my mother's eyes and saying, "I think I love you, but I'm so pissed at you that I can't tell anymore."

Talking has been especially difficult. Simple everyday communication is nearly impossible. My throat tightens and throbs. The clenched muscles remain unmoved by my pleas for an end to this most miserable trap of stifled speech. I wait for the day when this struggle will be over, but I am beginning to think that I am fooling myself. If I expect my voice to change, I'm going to be disappointed. Maybe if I let myself have these times of insecurity and doubt, I will learn to silence the incessant impatience of self-criticism. Maybe not.

I need to talk with Anne about my resistance to anti-depressants. I view taking them as a weakness, but is my need for them a greater weakness than my inability to speak? Perhaps my anxiety and depression are biochemical. If I had diabetes, would I refuse insulin? Why do I see this as a lack of courage? I fear that taking meds will numb my feelings. I am afraid they will inhibit me from completing the deeper soul-work I seek. I'm afraid of the possible side effects, but I also want to explore whether anti-depressants can decrease the anxiety and permit me to breathe more easily, thus paying the ransom on my voice, returning it to me.

I am concerned that Jane does not like the idea of me taking meds. She fears that I am looking for something that will fix that which is inherently unfixable, instead of dealing with the reality of my voice problem and accepting it. She believes the strangled speech will right itself when the reason for the clenching ceases, but I do not trust her assessment. I have been working diligently to excavate the emotional issues around this intense anxiety. Why do I have to continue to do it the hard way? Maybe just this once I don't have to be perfect and tough it out. Be strong. Endure. Such old, old patterns for me. This struggle has taken its toll. If that means I have failed, that I am not strong enough to take it, then I'll own that. Maybe the real weakness is to continue to keep batting my head against my own resistance and not explore other options.

It is clear to me that worrying about what others think is a sure sign that I need to back up and trust myself. Nobody else—

not Anne, not Beth, not even Jane—can know how hellish it has been for me. I'm going to approach the anti-depressant subject with Jane from a vantage point of strength. Position it as what I believe I need. Then I'm going to ask for her support from a place of empowerment and clarity instead of weakness and fear.

The part of me that fears Jane has very little to do with her. At a young age, I learned to defer to strong-minded people—especially strong-minded women—especially women with whom I am in close personal relationship. It is difficult for me to speak my mind. I fear disapproval and cringe at the slightest hint of abandonment. I fear that Jane will withdraw affection if I am angry with her or challenge her views. I try to decipher what is safe and what isn't. It's crazy, and all too familiar.

One remedy is to be self-referential, so that I don't buckle under and acquiesce to what others think is best, even if I don't feel that it is also right for me—especially as Jane doesn't ask for that. It's a terribly tough practice for me, and it's worse this year due to the lack of overall support I have often felt from Jane. She has been overwhelmed with work and the stress that my emotional healing process places on our relationship. In many ways, she is as depleted as I am. There has been disconnection between us. I feel less willing to open my heart and allow her to witness the terrors that hide inside. I feel lonely.

I try to trust the bigger picture. This is merely a transition, a hard time for both of us together, and for each of us individually. I wonder if maybe she isn't over in her own corner feeling just as disconnected as I am, wishing I'd be more supportive of her. Then I think about giving her attention, affection, sharing time together —all the things I want from her. I remember relationships take work and that they, too, have a flux and rhythm all their own, a contracting and an opening. We both need to slow down, nurture our selves. Be quiet. Heal.

Later in the week, we came to a sort of truce around the medication issue. Jane reaffirmed that her concern about the drugs is that they will have harmful side effects or that I might become addicted to them, but she also told me that she'd support me in exploring this option. I promised to get more information about anti-depressants before I rushed into it. I acknowledged that I am up against an edge that is overwhelming. Jane agreed that it has been emotionally draining for a long time and it doesn't seem to be getting easier. Maybe the meds will help.

I dreamt I was flying above the street in front of my childhood home, trying to escape people who were chasing me. The pursuers tried to grab my legs to pull me to the ground, but I settled in the high, caramel-smooth branches of a barren tree adjacent to the driveway. I managed to flee from every danger, even though I still felt a twinge of fear and panic. I was able to use my resources and my wits to get to safety.

In a separate dream, I was restoring several frescos, one of which depicted a painful, horribly traumatic tale on its surface layer. As I gently worked to remove the dirt and grime, I uncovered a rich, full story of happiness beneath. My collaborators and I decided to remove the entire outer stratum to reveal the peaceful story concealed under the faux top.

Chapter 21

In August of 1996, I traveled to Abiquiu, New Mexico to attend a five-day workshop with Clarissa Pinkola Estés, author of *Women Who Run with the Wolves*, at the Presbyterian Church's retreat facilities at Ghost Ranch. I hoped to recharge there, to be a reservoir as I listened to Dr. Estés, and allow her words to soothe my troubled heart. Because of my unreliable voice, however, I did not look forward to interacting with or talking to the other two hundred and twenty participants.

At the opening, Dr. Estés spoke about the necessity of individuation, of separating from what the wider culture tells us we must do or be. By culture, she meant the larger society as well as the particular subsets into which we are born—i.e. Catholic, Italian, female, etc. She said we must allow ourselves to separate and detach from the societal/cultural expectations, so that we can more fully become who we are, who we were meant to be.

Dr. Estés asked us to think about what we loved to do when we were ten years old and compare that to what we loved most at our present age. Enjoyment does not immediately come to mind when I think of myself as a ten-year old. When I delve deeper, beyond the trauma and the pain, I remember that, as a child, I loved being outdoors. I also loved singing and playing "movie stars" with my girl friends. When I had alone time, I spent hours drawing dresses, skirts, and outfits, imagining I would someday be a fashion designer.

During her talk, Dr. Estés reminded us that there is a price to pay for individuation. I agreed, but is the cost more than we pay for keeping silent? I have a broken voice. Was this part of my cost? Maybe my tense speech is a remnant of the fear-price.

Fear was alive and well during this retreat. It took up residence inside my belly. I didn't speak with many of the other retreat-goers. I was quite the turtle, cautiously shy. I struggled with letting that be okay. I tried to accept and embrace the quiet, but it was difficult. Very few of the other participants observed the sotto voce—the times of quiet and refection—requested at the start of the workshop. This became especially hard for me at meal times. I kept telling myself that it was okay to decline when people asked to sit by me or when they attempted to converse while standing in the serving line at the cafeteria. It was hard to not feel like the resident pariah.

One morning, as I walked to breakfast, it occurred to me that my lesson might be to try to accept myself—and my voice—as it was, at any given moment. I chose this retreat for the silence and the gifts of Dr. Estés. I didn't have to chat if I did not wish to do so. I was beholden to no one. If I didn't follow through on my self-imposed silence, I could blame only myself. Sotto voce aside, it was physically difficult for me to speak. The muscles in my neck ached from the effort. And always, I feared that my strangled speech would betray me—reveal that I was wounded and unable to mask my scars in a public setting. A loneliness surfaced during my days at Ghost Ranch that had nothing to do with the silence I had chosen, the sotto voce I craved.

What was I being invited to learn from each of these silences —chosen or not? Patience. Acceptance. I needed to be still in order to heal. I didn't fully understand why. I just knew that this was true, and I had to respect my right to it, even if all of the other attendees chatted their brains out and judged me as anti-social or withdrawn. I *was* sad and withdrawn.

The frustration I felt erupted in tears one afternoon, early on in my stay, as I sat alone by the dry riverbed behind the art building. I drew an oil pastel sketch of grief-stricken faces, masks with mournful eyes, thick, down-turned mouths. As my hand moved over the paper I began to understand that once I grew comfortable with the solitude and the silence it wouldn't matter what others thought or felt or wanted of me. I could put myself first.

The longer I stayed at Ghost Ranch, the more I became sated by the sights of the incredible mesas and the smells of the fresh, high-country piñon, juniper mornings. The healing power of nature was not a cliché to my sad and weary soul; it was profound medicine. It rained one night. Big winds etched puddles in the dusty clay. On the way back from the community gathering, lightning illuminated the sky over Camel Mesa. First a crackling noise, followed by a *kapow*, then electricity streaked through the inky darkness, magnetizing Camel Mesa. The high red rocks shimmered brightly against the startled night sky. When the light receded, the mesa melted into the dark while nearby hills remained etched with subtle luminescence, as if they had collected the day's heat and reflected it back in a slow, low glow.

The next morning, pink-tinged clouds hung over coral, rose, and sand-ribboned hills. And, oh the light! How it shook the air awake, how it shimmered around the edges of the mesas. Each day, I would feel drunk on the full, heady smell of piñon and rain-soaked clay. The dusty, sun-drenched hills fed me. They were dotted with sage-green, gray-green, brown, and umber brush, as thick as a slice of Italian bread.

One morning early in my stay at Ghost Ranch, I ached to phone Jane, to ease the isolation I felt, but I didn't call her, and I was glad that I waited. My urge arose from trying to take the edge off my loneliness, to touch something familiar and talk to someone who loved me, regardless of whether my words emerged in mangled consonants. I desperately wanted to get ground under my feet, to feel safer. I didn't feel comfortable in my skin. And I could not find a place on the conference grounds where I could fully relax. I carried a massive bundle of restlessness into this sacred place. Thankfully, the earth and the rain and the sky reminded me that there was much in this world that was far bigger than my own, individual angst. Somehow that truth calmed me.

Every day as I walked the grounds or hiked the hills around Ghost Ranch I was reminded, too, that there are a million little details that I overlook when I don't pay attention. I stooped to investigate a squashed beetle, its hard shell flattened into the dirt path. A swarm of ants feasted on the bug's legs and innards. The tasseled grasses waved to the cacti. Many dramas unfold below eye level—beetles and ants skittered about, rabbits scurried through tall grasses, small birds flitted through the air. Tiny orange, blue, and yellow wildflowers homesteaded those hills. People said there were snakes, scorpions, and coyotes, but I didn't see or hear any. Above eye level, a blue jay soared past. I captured the blue expanse of its wing in the corner of my eye and smiled, a deeply blue, deeply reverent smile.

One afternoon, I hiked into Box Canyon. Alongside a small stream I walked, crunching twigs underfoot, stepping over small rocks along the way, breathing in the cool air of the wooded lane I traveled. When at last I reached the path's end, I lay on the cool, hard rock at the mouth of the canyon and gazed into the vibrant sky. I felt as if I were flying, soaring up and away amid the pink and tan striated cliffs. In my mind's eye, I floated between two skinny pines and danced along the tiara of sky and clouds that crowned their delicate green spires. I listened to the wind. And prayed. I knew I was long-overdue for a chat with Mother Earth. I needed her advice. In that holy place, I felt more ready to receive it and to heed it.

My solitude at Ghost Ranch was balanced by large and small group gatherings. At those times, we retreat-goers would come together and try to untangle the conundrum of individuation. Each day, we broke into small groups and held sessions in which we discussed our responses to some of the questions that Dr. Estés had posed at the larger group gatherings. In one such small group session, I listened as people shared stories of their childhood. Nearly every woman in the room cried and told tales of pain and sorrow. Their words were balm to me. I realized that what I write *is* necessary. The cost to me personally has been high—in terms of my voice—but I have been given the ability to articulate, in words on paper, a child's experience of trauma. Perhaps, in some small way, my work could help other survivors, as well as me, feel less alone, less crazy.

In that room that afternoon, we women also shared stories about the things that we cherished when we were ten. I have come to realize that what I loved most at that age has resurfaced somehow in my adult life, in spite of every attempt to thwart me or break my stamina. It amazed me that I was able to excavate the spark that fueled my ten-year-old's heart and live an adult life as an artist and a writer. It hasn't been easy. It hasn't been linear. But I did it. It's important to honor that. I have been able to piece together enough fragments of my ten-year-old's splintered soul to salvage my art. That changes *everything*.

I unexpectedly visited a place of inner strength at Ghost Ranch—a place that I had wandered away from during the past few months of hard therapy. I desperately needed to connect with that resource, that sense of infinite wholeness—always our Truest Selves when we can see it. My challenge remains to accept my truth without shrinking. My art takes me deep into my history, but I have no real future without it. I can stay numb, or I can speak through my writing and through my clay sculptures and oil pastels.

I read May Sarton's *Journal of a Solitude*. In it, she writes about her depression and her anxiety, about creative tension and the need for solitude and silence. She bemoans how much energy it takes to be with people. She calls it a *collision*. She confesses self-doubt. Underneath her words lives a relentless belief in and trust of the rich, essential necessity of it all. Feeling. Being. Listening.

Sarton writes eloquently of her lifelong struggle with anger and unresolved conflict. She asks herself, "Will I ever grow up?" My heart reeled as I read her words. I recognized my own struggles in nearly every sentence. Pema Chödrön writes that a person's neurosis is her gold mine. Therapy isn't going to make my neuroses disappear. It's going to teach me a way to come to balance, so I can delve into the depths and retrieve whatever waits there.

Sarton's book rejuvenated me. I wanted to laugh and cry, dance and sing. Epiphany is not too strong a word for the sudden realization that I was not sick. I was not broken. I was a person who is doing the best she could to muddle through, just like every one else on this planet. The moodiness, the deep pain were tributaries from the Source, my creative channels, my passageways. Joy was a channel, too. I prayed that I could hold on to that clarity of feeling, that glorious understanding!

For a long time, I misnamed my sensitivity, my intuitive abilities as character defects. Slowly, I am coming to know that I am not weak, psychotic, or broken. I am caring, insightful, and creative. I can also be shy and withdrawn, easily overwhelmed, and emotionally confused. But knowing this, being able to identify the strengths and the encumbrances that are part of who I am, is different from categorically dismissing myself as too touchy, too needy, too weak, too sensitive.

Through my writing, I choose to be naked in the world. Balance and boundaries are called for, to ease the discomfort that is inherent in the telling. I need to learn how to regulate these. So I can take better care of my sensitive heart, so I do not get trampled, so I do not spiral into a wicked trap of self-recrimination.

In her mid-week evening talk, Dr. Estés noted that people grow on sinew and bone, not on sugar or sweetness. How ironic that, in our culture, we are taught to think that challenges and sorrows are the enemy, derailing us from our rightful happiness. Loss of innocence is a rite of passage in which we learn that the world isn't perfect and good. Without this awareness, we never learn to protect ourselves. According to Dr. Estés, this rite of passage is initiated to re-heal and re-vive the injured, maimed parts of the Spirit, so that we may fulfill our life's purpose. One's purpose doesn't have to be as grand as growing up to be the President of the United States or a Nobel Laureate. It can be as simple and as valuable as being a good parent, a caring teacher, a grower of good fruits and vegetables.

To identify one's life purpose one must feed one's Instinctual Nature. Pure symbolic language—art, literature, music, stories, etc.—sustains Instinctual Nature. Sorrow cannot kill this natural essence. Grief won't kill it, either. Abuse can silence it for a time, cage it, stomp on it, contain it, belittle it. Our job as human beings is to silence the Ego's *my way or the highway* attitude. Ego is meant to *follow* Soul and Spirit, not blaze the trail. Dr. Estés believes that moderation is key in our efforts to nurture our Instinctual Nature, but she redefines moderation as liberal, juicy, generous, sexy, wonderful—measured out to last and last.

When I called Jane later in the week, there was nothing juicy, generous, or wonderful in my attempts to convey to her all that I have been learning about myself. My throat clenched, my voice tightened. I felt inadequate—frustrated, silenced *again*. Even in the midst of all this potent Ghost Ranch medicine, my wound is very deep. It is primal, visceral, non-verbal. Is it my Instinctual Nature trying to be heard? This inability to talk without struggle drags my Ego to its knees. I am ready to cry uncle and give up.

I know I am my own worst enemy. In my family of origin, in my birth culture, I was not supposed to grow to be a separate individual. I have hit granite with the essential validity of who I am in the world. Do I have a right to exist? Can I trust it? I must continue to kill the internalized parent that tells me I can't be separate from my mother, my father, my siblings; can't tell *my* truth. Somehow I saved a glowing ember of consciousness for later, for now, for the time in my adulthood when I could make good use of it. My Instinctual Nature refuses to roll over and die, even in the face of extreme assault.

That is why my painting and clay sculpting are essential, and my dreams, too. The symbolic language of my subconscious actively guides me. The process continues even when I can't express myself in traditional ways—like talking.

At one of our nightly large group gatherings, Dr. Estés asked us to imagine ourselves standing beside a river carrying a bundled load. She implored us to look inside the bundle and name the contents that weighed us down, hindering us from fording the river and continuing on our life's path.

And what is my load? *Mother-anger*. It keeps me from crossing over. When I shared this with the women in my small group, the next day, my cheeks burned.

After lunch, I felt a strong urge to move my body and escape the confines of hallways filled with talking people. I hiked Chimney Rock mesa. I tried to forgive myself for ratting on my mother during the small group session. I struggled, too, with still being unable to connect with fellow conference-goers. At lunch, I shied away from someone who asked to share my table. On Chimney Rock, I reminded myself that I am courageous to have come to Ghost Ranch—me, a person prone to anxiety attacks, me an introvert with a voice problem, coming by myself to a retreat with over two hundred strangers. I was either totally out of my mind, or one of the bravest people I know.

Later, Dr. Estés talked of a period of dissolution, a time of profound loneliness, of waiting in the dark. She said it was like sitting in a vat of dissolving solution. One must stay in the cook pot until all the old flesh falls off the bone. I found myself nodding, intimately aware of how the hot, searing dissolution liquid felt against my tender skin. Sitting in the stew pot requires great sacrifice. Great patience. Great fortitude. One must relinquish all that stands in the way—even the things that one loves—if these things become an obstacle, a thief of one's precious time. Dr. Estés encouraged each of us to ask questions and explore our subconscious through art and dreams. After the solitude, after the solo, internal work, after it all comes to fruition, she said that we would return renewed and refreshed, better able to bring wholeness to others through example, through teaching, through support, and through thanksgiving.

"You have to tell the truth for the Psyche to move on," Dr. Estés reminded us. Her words affirmed that my struggle to name my truths is not foolhardy. It's okay to be messy, to be confused, inchoate, but I needed to learn to ask for help. Once, being a *good girl* helped me survive. It was now time to lay down that burden and be a girl who says *No* to others and *Yes* to herself. To give myself permission to be a girl who isn't always nice, a girl who is sometimes cranky, snarly—maybe even bitchy. Fiercer. I need to learn how to be fiercer and create a larger circle around me, generously buffered with room to expand. I need to *receive* as well as give.

I buried Good Girl Saracino yesterday, back behind Kitchen Mesa at Ghost Ranch. I drew a picture of a gravestone inscribed with the words: Good Girl Saracino 1954-1996. I left her there among the mesas and the cottonwoods to rest for eternity in this glorious place. She deserves a reprieve. She has worked hard; she has given so much of herself. It's time she receives something in return.

Later that day, I decided to resurrect Good Girl Saracino and *retire* her—not bury her. I set her up in a cabin at Ghost Ranch. I gave her a pension, a room of her own, and a four-wheel-drive vehicle, so she could go anywhere she wanted. She would receive three meals a day in the Ghost Ranch cafeteria, and she didn't ever have to do the dishes. She could spend the rest of her life soaking up the mesas and the electric blue sky. She's earned her rest.

Chapter 22

Jane, our friend Nina, and I heard Pema Chödrön speak at the First Unitarian Universalist Church in San Francisco on a balmy September evening. It was good to finally see our longtime mentor in person. Pema didn't cover any material unfamiliar to us, but her wisdom still remained rich and textured. Each time I listen to a cassette tape of one of her talks or read from one of her many books on loving-kindness and Tibetan Buddhism, I understand her teachings at a different level. It is clear from her writing and her talks that she embraces her human limitations and tries to be compassionate toward her neuroses and attachments. And because she does, she inspires me.

During the question-and-answer period, that evening in San Francisco, a man relayed an experience he had in which he witnessed a mother hitting her child on a street corner. The episode triggered the man's own painful past, filling him with great rage. He told Pema and the audience that he had yelled at the woman until the cops came and arrested her. He asked Pema how to handle the anger he felt toward people who have children without first attending to their own wounds.

Pema's answer was simple, yet difficult. She told him, "Start with yourself. Know your own anger. Come to know it and have compassion for it and the rest will most likely take care of itself. Because your heart and mind will gradually soften over time, and while you won't eradicate the anger, you will know it and perhaps not go to a hard place with it as often. Let it be in a different way. That's when a shift can occur. You don't let it go as much as you let it be. You disarm the need to be hard with it. You come to know it as just a feeling, without judging it or condemning it. You aren't overwhelmed by it either."

Pema's words touched my sore spots. From experience I, too, have found that I can soften my response to my hard emotions by *feeling* them. We humans need to pay attention to our personal wounds so we don't end up abusing our "kids"—whether that be our actual biological children, our internal child, our spouses, our co-workers, or our friends and family. The woman with the child is a reminder of what can happen if we do not take this critical responsibility to heart.

After the Pema Chödrön retreat, Jane and I drove south to Monterey. We spent the afternoon strolling around Cannery Row before trying to find the Days Inn in Carmel. The map we had offered an overview of the area, but omitted the finer details of side streets. I grew grouchy because my voice tightened every time

I tried to be Jane's co-pilot, navigating our way. Later, as I stewed over my defective voice and how impotent it made me feel, I realized that I needed to grieve the loss of easy speech, just as surely as I would have needed to grieve the loss of an arm or a leg or an eye. An essential part of me is impaired. If I let myself acknowledge the loss instead of minimizing it, I will be better able to accept the disability. Lord knows, I can't bargain with these clenched vocal muscles. Magical thinking doesn't help. The situation is one-hundred percent out of my control.

The next morning, we drove to Big Sur and walked along the shore for nearly two hours. The waves crashed against the towering rock formations as surfers glided on the surface only to be toppled by swells of curled water. Jane took pictures of the ocean, the trees, and the beach. I sang *Amazing Grace* to the gigantic Pacific—even yelled to release the tension in my throat and my diaphragm. My singing isn't worth shit these days. My voice cracks and what once was effortless is now cramped.

That night before I fell asleep, I asked my Soul for information about how to cope with my voice, what to expect, and how to accept what is.

I dreamt that I was writing a newspaper article on a local woman who was a psychic/healer and had arranged to be invited to a party at this woman's house. At the party, the Healer placed her hands on my arms, my legs, and my belly. I was conscious throughout the treatment—which was considered rare and a sign of deeper healing. I grieved, feeling a full, deep range of emotions without manifesting these outwardly. After the treatment I gradually returned to full consciousness. I began singing loudly. My voice was clear and strong. I felt immensely happy.

After we returned home to Minneapolis, I felt insecure about my ability to sustain myself through work projects and the day-to-day stresses of just plain living. I grew anxious about being anxious, and it spiraled into one huge angst fest. Maybe there is a medical reason for my inability to speak. Maybe it isn't just all in my head. Maybe I have a thyroid condition. Or maybe it's early onset of menopause, as my voice tension exacerbates around my menstrual cycle. Maybe I've inherited a defective gene; my grandfather died of Multiple Lateral Sclerosis—a disease that eroded his muscles. Maybe this whole situation is a neurological disorder—and my synapses are misfiring. However, it isn't constant. There are times when my speech is fine.

I dreamt last night that Anne rocked me and I cried in her arms. In the dream, I wasn't completely comfortable with her holding me. I needed nurturing, but it was hard to let it in.

In therapy this week I mustered the courage to tell Anne that I felt frustrated. I've tried hard to let go of my expectations and accept my voice as it is. But I can't. It matters a great deal to me that I can't talk. It matters that every second of my waking day I am anxious about whether or not my voice is going to give out. It shatters my confidence. It keeps me from engaging with people, from communication and connection. I have so much to say, and I can't say any of it. I sobbed through the session.

I have hit bottom. I sobbed during my Hakomi session this week, too, leaving rings of snot and tears on Beth's bodywork table linens. She sat beside me and held my hand. She encouraged me to keep writing and doing my artwork because I find strength in these. When I try to speak, I feel like a failure, but what is inside me emerges with ease when I write, draw, paint and sculpt.

In my attempt to find a way to quell this raging anxiety, I

decided to take Gingko and St. John's Wort capsules. A holistic doctor, in *Natural Health* magazine, recommended these as alternatives to Western anti-depressants and anti-anxiety medication. It might be the placebo effect, but I feel less mired in the muck.

Anne had suggested a doctor for me to call about a medication consultation, and I called him and left a message. I'm glad I finally took this step. I don't have to be the tough little soldier anymore. The Good Girl who doesn't complain, just endures, is safely retired at Ghost Ranch. I need all the support I can muster. My body is extremely tired. So is my Spirit. How much humiliation and shame do I have to endure before I say enough is enough?

Anne told me that she thought that by now, with all the significant emotional work I have done with her, I would have shown some evidence of regaining my voice, but it hasn't improved. The speech therapy didn't help. Voice lessons didn't help. Hakomi hasn't helped. Neither have the Chinese anti-anxiety herbs or the Valerian root pills. Nothing has eased the stranglehold on my normal voice.

I talked with Jane about my upcoming medication consultation. It is clear that we still don't fully agree on the subject. After supper, she left for a class, and I cried on and off for the rest of the evening. This is one of the hardest places I've ever been in my life, and one of the most difficult decisions I have had to make. It's *my* life, *my* problem. I need Jane's support, and I am angry that it is not readily forthcoming. I feel abandoned.

Jane is concerned about side effects and worried that I am putting all my hopes into these pills. She doesn't want me to be hurt by the meds. She is also coming from a place of fear about how anti-depressants affect people. I can't let her uneasiness deter me. Maybe the deeper truth for me is to trust Jane's love and support even though it doesn't look (or feel) like what I need right now.

The doctor we met with was very kind and easy to be around, but it was still hard for me to talk with him. He asked questions and I had to answer, which meant I had to speak. My voice tightened, which enabled him to see and hear, first-hand, the reason for our meeting. I fidgeted and cried. I told him I was at the end of my rope. I tried to explain how anxious I get at the most insignificant things, such as talking on the phone with strangers *and* with friends. I told him I was withdrawing from life because it was too hard to talk. I told him all the routes I have taken up to this point to address my situation—to no avail.

He asked me if I had experienced dizziness? Tingling? Loss of balance? Blurred vision? Numbness? He was trying to ascertain whether I had MS or some other neurological condition. I told him my condition was pretty much confined to tightness in my throat and diaphragm. He said he thought I had a panic/anxiety disorder. He felt I had an eighty-percent chance of being helped by medication.

He explained the various kinds of anti-depressant and anti-anxiety medications and their side effects. He responded respect-fully to Jane's questions and concerns. He told us he would recommend Paxil for me because of its ability to treat both depression and anxiety without the harmful side effects of other, stronger anti-anxiety drugs such as Valium and Busbar.

Afterward, as Jane drove us home she reached over and held my hand. She said she would support me if I decided to try the medication. I squeezed her hand in response and nodded before I burst into tears, relieved by her support. We have both had to re-examine our assumptions and judgments about anti-depressants. It felt good to know that Jane had found a sort of peace with this option. Later at home, we e-mailed our friend Berna, who is a pharmacist, and asked her to send us information on Paxil. It was a big step in a much-needed direction.

When I took my first dose of Paxil, it felt strange, but I urged myself not to freak out. I lay in bed thinking about the little yellow pill inside me releasing its synthetic biochemicals. I tried to trust that it was doing its job. I reminded myself that it would take up to four weeks for the medication to manifest itself in my body. I shouldn't worry if I didn't experience positive effects right away.

Maybe my voice is on its way home. I can hardly wait!

Today is the twenty-ninth anniversary of the day we left Seneca Falls. Next year I want to gather friends to officially honor the thirtieth anniversary. It is my hope to have put this wrenching leave-taking in the past by then, to release its hold over me. I am close to that point.

I took my third dose of Paxil last night. So far I can't tell if anything is working. I still have trouble talking, but there has been a subtle shift in my internal system. The edge is lessening— not a lot yet, but some. The internal fire is not quite as fierce. My mood is beginning to lift and lighten.

Even with the Paxil, I stumbled through a phone conversation with my mother this week. She asked if Jane and I wanted to drop by to watch the Vikings football game on their big screen TV. I declined her offer. I don't blame her for trying. I know she misses me. I miss her, too, but there have been too many traumas, too much drama, too much smothering. We've both hurt one another. I know I've injured her by trying to evade her grasp in order to create my own life. I hope someday I can come to reconciliation. Maybe then I'd feel better able to see my mother on a regular basis. For now, that will have to wait.

I turn forty-two on Friday. My, my, I am getting older. Wiser? Only time will tell. We cleaned the basement this weekend, and I ran across old journals from college and from graduate school. Even then, I was writing about my search for authenticity. It's nice to know some glimmer of life was inside me, seeking its rightful path, even way back then.

Maybe I was emboldened by the Paxil, but this week I confessed to Jane that sometimes things feel so hard I just want to die. She cried and confided that she felt scared and sad. This emotional roller coaster I have been riding has been too hard for too long. She didn't know if she had the energy to keep going. I didn't seem to be getting any better. She felt as if there wasn't enough room in our relationship for her feelings. My energy was too dark and heavy. She thought we needed more balance, more playfulness. She said that maybe staying in therapy wasn't the answer. She suggested that perhaps I was stuck. Maybe I have been in therapy so long because the feeling and the pain were familiar to me; it's what I knew.

We both cried. I felt as if my therapy and my need to heal were wrecking my relationship. I tried to listen, tried to hear and accept the good points she made, but I don't think ending therapy is the answer. I can lessen the intensity by alternating my psychotherapy and my Hakomi sessions, and by confining my emotional work to the time allotted for each. I can consciously seek out play and recreation to bring levity to my life.

Maybe there is a more playful way to let go of my anger. I don't want to lose Jane. I don't want to hurt her. I do want to consider her comments. Some of them are truthful and insightful; some of them arise from her personal process of transition and the ways in which it bumps against mine. Maybe the Paxil will help, after it kicks in full force. Maybe it will even out my moods.

Joy is possible. If I can bring gratitude (when I am able to access it) to the process, I might just be able to lift this heaviness.

170

Here's the joyful part: I survived.

I want that child I once was to know that we made it. I want to give her a sense of hope that no matter how hard and awful things were, somehow, we survived. Spirit never deserted us, even though plenty of other people did. All is not doom and gloom. All is not lost. Maybe that's what that scared kid inside me needs to hear. She isn't a hopeless case. She is going to grow up to be a fine woman—one who managed to salvage the spark of her essential authenticity and carry it through the muck and mire to higher ground.

I *am* more than my experiences, more than the trauma, more than the fear and the grief and the anger. I have an essential goodness that wasn't damaged. It's longing to shine forth. I get to be happy, now. I deserve it.

I'm up to twenty milligrams of Paxil, and I can definitely feel the jitteriness.

In my Hakomi session, Beth and I talked about play and how crucial it is to my healing. This is quite the challenge for an overly responsible six-year-old. Beth suggested that if that inner kid needed to feel responsible about something, she could focus on playing. Her job is to be curious and inquisitive, meandering and non-task oriented. Bubble baths, leaf collecting, bubbles, jacks, reading storybooks, making snow angels, watching the clouds, laughing—those are my healing tools.

Beth is right, of course. I am too driven, too focused, too intense, too wired. And my nervous system is already tightly wound—partly as a result of heredity, and partly in response to the high-voltage surge of external stimuli I encountered in my family as it was falling apart all around me when I was a child.

The Paxil continues to be a hard adjustment. At first, I felt only a slight headache and tingly hands—too much energy? The headaches went away, and then I had a hard time sleeping. I'd wake at three or four in the morning—which, for me, is quite unusual. The twenty-milligram dose also makes me tremble a bit. I feel nauseated. Sometimes I get a gagging reflex in my throat. It goes away with a sip of water, so I think it's connected to the dry mouth I've been experiencing. I woke with shaky hands one morning. Sometimes when I yawn, I feel tremors in my hamstrings. Hopefully some (or all) of these side effects will dissipate as my body grows accustomed to the drug.

Is all this worth it?

Balance is a sign of good boundaries.

Anne told me about an article she read, which noted that it is important to honor one's "woundedness" without acquiring it as one's identity. She told me she felt she could be better about honoring my successes, my strengths, and the breakthroughs I've made in order to help give me a greater sense of confidence and power. I told her I wanted to get the message across to the scared girl inside me that she grew up to be a woman who is successful, a woman who has good friends, work she likes, enough money, and a loving relationship. I wanted her to know that things are going to work out; she's going to be okay.

How long I have distanced myself from the scared girl I once was in order to accomplish the goals I set for myself in my adult life! I cringe at identifying with what I saw as my defects—the small girl hiding in the shadows. I didn't want to accept her as part of my adult self.

Today, I make a promise to that fragile child. *I will honor your anger and your ability to tell the truth. And I will make room for play.*

It's been two weeks since my first dose of Paxil. I've been feeling fairly stable, in spite of the fact that I am very busy with freelance writing projects. The excruciating anxiety is lessening. I no longer feel as if my insides are prickly with angst. I still get nervous, especially when I talk to my friends about personal, emotional stuff, but the weight of it is less than it used to be. Overall I am able to take deeper, fuller breaths.

I still feel tired, although it's not the same bone-aching tiredness I felt this summer before I started taking Paxil. Then, I felt completely drained, unable to keep going. Yet, as much as my fatigue has lessened, my voice still hasn't returned in full force. It's been three weeks and my need to crawl out of my skin has lessened, but I am beginning to think that maybe the medication won't bring my voice back.

In therapy this week, my voice refused to cooperate. I withdrew in frustration and refused to speak. Anne asked me how old I was feeling at that moment. I replied, "Six." She handed me a pad of paper and a pen and told me to write or draw whatever that six-year-old needed to say. I opened the pen cap and stared at the blank paper trying to conjure courage. Eventually, I took the pen and scrawled thick, black marks across the page. The pen died, and I ripped the paper and threw it on the floor. Anne offered me a pillow to hit. I wanted to punch it, but I felt foolish doing so in front of her. I also felt afraid that she might reprimand me. Eventually, my urge to smack won out. I whacked the pillow and stomped my foot.

An urge to yell surfaced, but I squelched it. I felt self-conscious about ranting in front of Anne. She suggested that she could either yell with me or leave the room and let me scream by myself. I couldn't bear the thought of her leaving the room. On the count of three, we yelled together. I was amazed. It felt so damned good.

I'm up to thirty milligrams of Paxil a day. The doctor said that the typical dosage is twenty to thirty milligrams for depression. For anxiety, the typical dosage is forty to sixty milligrams. I hope the side effects stay manageable.

I don't know if it's the Paxil, the therapy, the bodywork—or all three—but something is opening up. I screamed twice this week. I pounded the big red ball during my Hakomi session. I am doing well with my intention to face whatever is present. I am even managing to be more playful in my day-to-day life. I still harbor a lot of rage and sadness. All my feelings of self-abandonment are surfacing as well. I cringe to think of how I disowned my wounds so I could function in the adult world. It's time to gather the hurt parts and return them to the fold. That sweet girl I once was is more than her miserable past. And so am I. Hope is returning. Life is good. It can be hard and messy, but it is good, too. It's okay to feel joy.

1997

Chapter 23

I am thinking seriously about inviting my mother to a joint therapy session. I have been trapped in the ingrained belief that I have no right to a voice in my family. This emotional tangle is covert most of the time, making it difficult for me to name, but I am ready now to focus on what I want to say to Mom and how I want to say it. I am angry and I need to make room for this powerful self-defining piece that I was denied as a child.

It is ironic—given the subsequent emotional fallout I experienced from having written *No Matter What*—that I felt most powerful the first time I read my work in front of an audience. In

1991, two years before the onset of the first signs of my voice problems, I was one of four fiction writers who participated in the Minneapolis-based Loft Mentor Series. Each of us "mentees," as we called ourselves, read our work as a front act for one of four nationally acclaimed visiting writers who were our mentors in the program. I was one of two writers who opened for Native American poet and writer Barney Bush.

The evening of the reading, I paced backstage trying to walk off mounting anxiety. Knowing this was the first time I had ever read in front of a public audience, Barney Bush advised me to forget about my ego and tap into the passion that led me to write in the first place. I took a deep breath and walked on stage. The first face my eyes landed upon was my mother's. My heart screamed, *You can't read THIS out loud with her in the room. Everyone will KNOW!*

Somehow, I managed to calm myself and read part of what would later become the first chapter of *No Matter What*. Halfway down the opening page, I found my confidence and relaxed. I read with a passionate, clear voice. During the post-reading reception, people told me I had great stage presence. These are words I can hardly comprehend, now.

Perhaps after I muster the courage to say the difficult things I need to say to my mother in a therapy session, my physical voice will return as well. Even if it doesn't, I know I will be able to reclaim my emotional voice.

I want to be honest with my mother, for possibly the first time in my life. She has never read *No Matter What*. She says the novel conjures things she would rather not think about. It's a painful book. I know that. It was painful to write.

Why do I need to confront my mother to her face? I can scream at empty chairs and pound pillows and shout at the wall to alleviate some of my anger, but it is not enough. The damage calls for more drastic measures, and bringing Mom into a therapy session is definitely a drastic measure. It's subversive. It's also exhilarating. I need the visceral experience of breaking the silence between us. My body needs to feel the power of my truth in my mouth in her presence.

I want to directly and compassionately relate my truth to Mom without shaming or blaming her. I also want to put the responsibility squarely where it belongs—on her shoulders, not mine. I'm responsible for cleaning my own house, grappling with the impact that our relationship continues to have on my life, but the innumerable ways that she failed me as a mother belong to her. Maybe in some small way, our joint meeting will contribute to her healing as well.

Jane and I are house-sitting in Albuquerque, New Mexico for a month. My dream of being a snowbird has come true. For the last five years, Jane and I have been talking about moving out of Minnesota. That's part of our reason for this month away. We want to see if Albuquerque is a place to which we might relocate.

Here in this land of balmy winters, I work on rewriting chapters of my sequel, tightening the action, and polishing the dialogue. The character development is going much more smoothly, especially with regards to Grace. I needed to give her more depth, make her multi-dimensional, give the reader a reason to believe that she would take in two lost little girls on a rainy night and feed and shelter them. Grace's compassion and love for Regina and Rosa sutures their broken hearts enough to enable them to return to their mother. That's Grace's role in the book. She guides and protects Regina and Rosa because their own mother isn't capable of it.

It's strange to be writing of a mother-guide even as I struggle with what I feel is lacking in my relationship with my own mother.

It's both a mirror and a reframing of what cannot exist between us. I've felt frustrated that my mother won't—perhaps can't—heal her own heart, at least attempt to do her part in resolving our schism. I worried that her inability to change would impede my ability to heal. Now I realize that I can finish my part even if hers remains unchanged. There are nine people in my family, which means that there are nine different truths, nine different points of view, each equally valid. I have a right—no, a responsibility—to name my truth and to grapple with it, integrate it into my life.

It feels so damn good to be writing again. No pressure about publishing or performing my work, just the pure joy of crafting the story, hearing the dialogue, creating the plot—it is Heaven! It's time to finish this sequel. I've been afraid of it for so long, worried that writing it would invite more trauma causing me to spiral again into something horrible and hard.

The places into which I delve in order to invoke what I need to say in a book can be frightening. After my first novel was published, and my voice began its slow and steady decline, I grew to fear my writing. I saw it as the root cause of my strangled speech, the thorn in the side of my attempts to reclaim my truth. There have been many times throughout the last four years when I identified my writing as the enemy. Still, part of me always knew that this was inaccurate, the foggy vision of a woman in pain. Writing is central to who I am, whether or not I'm ever published again, or am ever able to read my work in public. If I stopped writing, I would wither. It's the worst kind of hell to be fearful of what is so essential.

Maybe geographical distance, like time, can help mend some of the residual fears that linger around my right to write. The physical distance between New Mexico and Minnesota blesses me with space to contemplate what I want and need. The New Mexico landscape pulls me out of context. It is so dissimilar to the landscape of Minnesota or of western New York state, where I grew up, that I am able to enter a different zone, a world in which I am just *me*, not somebody's daughter, not somebody's sister. Here in New Mexico, with ample geographical distance between my family and me, I gain a clearer psychological perspective. My deeply felt losses used to arise from the fact that my family was devastatingly torn apart. I am growing to realize that a different type of aching abides in me, as well. And this grief is for the young girl I used to be—for all of her abandoned hopes, for all her considerable fears.

One of the gifts of therapy has been to help me know that I am not alone. I no longer have to be a brave soldier on a solo mission—strong and enduring. There is strength in opening the sore spots to others, but how to choose which others to trust? Loyalty is a tricky thing in my Italian American family. I was raised to revere La Famiglia —to place it above all else, even my own sanity. In our household, there was no "I," no "Me," no "Mine," only the perpetual "We," "Us," "Ours," For years, I kept silent to remain loyal. That meant I had to betray myself. Now whenever possible, I scale the wall of secrecy and open my heart to Anne or Beth or Jane or a cherished friend. Doing so can be quite problematic, however. When I choose self-loyalty, shame and guilt rear their ferocious heads. At times the roar is weak. More often, it is deafening.

The long road back to me has been arduous, but necessary. The finger-pointing voices plague me, but they lessen with each story told, each truth reclaimed. Every year, I grow a sturdier, more affirming sense of Self. All my life I have needed to call upon great courage to battle the *big-family-guns*. I struggle to find the counterpoint balance where I can speak with clarity and kindness as well as with biting truth. Still the voices nag, *Who do you think you are to drag your mother through the muck and the mire?* Me, of all people. I am the one who tacitly agreed to shield Mom from her broken heart. What happens when I refuse to honor that sacred pact, when I close my heart to her grieving eyes? What happens when my own survival necessitates tyranny? Does this make me a bad daughter? A turncoat? Will my mother excommunicate me from her heart? Do I care?

Yes. I care.

I wish I could choose to love myself *and* my mother, but the old family pattern won't allow it. Confronting Mother breaks the ultimate family rule: don't hold a mirror up to Mom's life. Don't force her to reckon with the choices she has made. Don't drag her over the blistering coals. The past is the past. How long does she have to pay for her mistakes?

How long, indeed, do *I* have to pay for her mistakes?

I must discard the old rules; invent new ones. I choose not to protect Mom anymore. I abdicate that role. I may lose my mother's love as a consequence of this upcoming therapy session. I may not. In the end I will reclaim my right to a distinct and separate life.

And maybe even my voice.

In February, after Jane and I had returned to Minneapolis, I immediately began to miss the spaciousness I had felt in New Mexico, how opened I had been to my own vast internal landscape. New Mexico was good for my spirit. Jane and I both enjoyed a warmer January than we are used to and we took advantage of the opportunity to better acquaint ourselves with Albuquerque. We still aren't sure if we want to move there. We prefer Santa Fe, because it is smaller and less industrial-looking, but it's very expensive to live there. Time will tell where we will land.

Last week, I went to see Mia, a psychic whom Jane and I have visited many times over the past six years. She affirmed that 1996 had been a very hard year for me. She said I was stronger, now, more spiritually and creatively centered, independent and confident. I was ready to be successful. I felt deserving of it. She saw some conflict on the family level. She said someone was holding me back. She saw me breaking free of that and coming into my own.

After the reading, I told Mia that I was having my mother in for a therapy session. She said that would be very good for me. She had information from my grandmothers (both whom had passed). My mother's mother (who died when I was two) told Mia that my mother feels guilt about something she did, but she shuts down, and refuses to hear anything about it. Mia told me that Nonna said I needed to remember that I couldn't say anything to my mother that would be worse than what she already says to herself. Nonna would be in the therapy session with me. I would feel a chill and know she was present. Nonna told me not to take care of my mother, to tell the truth.

Then my voice will clear up.

I called my mother and asked if she would agree to come to therapy with me in March. She said, "Of course," then asked me what the session was about. I took a deep breath, gripped the back of my chair, and told her that I wanted to talk to her about our relationship. There were things I needed to tell her but I wanted to do so in a therapy session because I felt nervous.

"You shouldn't be nervous talking to your mother," she said.

"Well, I am," I replied.

I told her that I had arranged for a separate therapist to be at the session, just for her. I wanted her to feel safer. I said I would pay for that therapist as well as my own. I emphasized that my intention was not to shame her but to have a conversation. She said she didn't feel threatened. As long as there was love, we could face anything. I took her comment as a gift and a hopeful premonition for our upcoming meeting.

To prepare, I made a list of key points, which I planned to use as a reference in the session if I got sidetracked. I practiced reading this list out loud. Each time, I began by yelling the sentences. By the end of the list I was in tears.

On a bright, chilly March morning, I arrived at Anne's office fifteen minutes before my scheduled ten o'clock appointment, so I could have some prep time with my therapist before my mother arrived. Nella, the woman I had hired to be my mother's therapist, was there, too. After a quick review of what to expect in the session, I took a few minutes to create an altar of protection. I had asked Jane and my friends for small objects that I could take into the session with me. I wanted to feel their support even though they couldn't physically be in the room with me at this hardest of junctures. They would be present in spirit. I placed a cloth on the floor and set their mementos upon it. I invited Spirit to join me, to sustain me, to offer courage and comfort. I asked Nonna to stand beside me during the two-hour session. I was both terrified and exhilarated. This was the day it seems I had been waiting for my whole life.

My mother arrived at Anne's office on time, and we began our session. I started by thanking her for coming, applauding her courage. I told her I had tried for many years, in many ways, to have this conversation with her, but her tears had always silenced me. I laid out the tale of my life as her daughter, from my point of view. I spared nothing. I tried to be compassionate. I hope I succeeded. I won't ever fully know.

I told her that as a child I had wanted so much to take away the hurt and pain I saw in her eyes. I told her that as I grew older I learned to love her more than I loved myself. I thought that if I

184

could make her happier, she would see my pain and protect me. Instead, I became her confidante. I kept her secrets. I swallowed my own.

Throughout the session, I filled in the details relating concrete incidences of how and why I felt disconnected, abandoned, unloved, angry, and invisible. To my mother's credit, she listened and responded. The few times that she slipped into her safety net of wounded face and tears, Nella, the therapist I had hired to tend to Mom, came to her rescue (and mine). She comforted my mother and encouraged her to focus on her own feelings.

In closing, I told Mom that I was taking responsibility for my life and my childhood wounds. I emphasized that I was not trying to blame her. I understood that she did the best she could, given the circumstances of her life. I said that while blame wasn't called for, accountability was. She was my parent. She was responsible for nurturing me, helping me learn how to love and cherish myself, how to navigate in the world. It was her job to keep me safe. When I needed guidance, she didn't give it to me. When I needed protection, she didn't deliver. When I needed to grieve, there was no room.

I told her that I loved her, but I would no longer protect her at the cost of losing myself. I told her I didn't know if we could ever be truly close, but I hoped that we could find a way to connect that was more respectful and nurturing to each of us.

When I left Anne's office I felt exhausted, but strong and brave, free at last from holding back the terrible truth. I felt as if I had grown up in a deep and abiding way and had reclaimed my adulthood. The session with my mother was the most difficult thing I have ever done. And I survived. I am filling to the edges of my skin. What else in life could be more frightening than to assert myself to my mother's face and say, "I count. I choose me this time. I choose me!"

Chapter 24

I have requested that my mother and I communicate exclusively via e-mail. Despite the fact that we live only nineteen miles from one another, I feel safer interacting with her electronically rather than in person. Although it feels strange not to pick up the phone and call her or suggest that we meet for breakfast, e-mail gives me the precious distance I need to create a zone of protection. From this country called Online, I can traverse the distance that separates us and attempt to re-establish a workable mother-daughter relationship.

I feel emboldened and confident, ready to forge ahead in my determination to establish and maintain the boundaries between our lives. These demarcations are crucial if I am to survive intact and grow into the woman I'm meant to be. I'm saddened that it must be so, but resolved to accept the ground rules I established that day in Anne's office. I will not take care of my mother's pain at the cost of erasing my own reality. E-mail becomes a force field of bytes and bits, freeing me to express my thoughts and feelings without the immediate cause and effect of a face-to-face conversation. Within this cyber breathing space, I can inhale and exhale with ease, certain that my words won't be interrupted, erased, silenced, dismissed.

When I saw my family-practice doctor for my yearly check-up, I talked to her about my voice struggles. I filled her in on how long I had been grappling with this strangled speech—nearly four years, now. She listened quietly and when I had finished, she asked whether I was an incest survivor. I nodded and added that I was also working hard to resolve conflicts I had with my mother, with whom I felt I had no voice. We talked about how important therapy was, and she asked if I felt that my anti-anxiety meds were helping.

"Yes," I said, "Except they haven't improved my voice at all." To rule out a medical condition, she ordered a thyroid test, which came out negative. So, my speech concerns aren't physical?

Jane and I are getting more serious about leaving Minnesota. The idea of relocating has been percolating since January when we spent the month in New Mexico. We both want a respite from the harsh Midwestern winters, and Jane despises the humid, sticky Minnesota summers. We excluded Albuquerque from our list of destination options because the city's economy isn't conducive to either of our small businesses. And the climate is too hot for Jane. Now, instead, we are considering Colorado. We have friends who live in Denver, so up-rooting would be less traumatic.

We asked two of our Colorado friends for the name of their realtor and flew to Denver the first weekend in May to look at thirty properties. We hadn't officially told our Minneapolis friends that we were serious about a move out of state. We wanted to investigate Denver and see if it felt like a good match before we told them the news. It was eighty degrees and sunny during our sojourn in the mile-high city. The downtown skyline of brick and glass shimmered against the breathtaking backdrop of mountains and sky. Parks and pathways were nestled among neighborhoods. Creeks and lakes meandered through the cityscape. By the weekend's close, we decided that this menagerie of urban bustle and natural beauty held the promise of home.

Back in Minneapolis, we reviewed all the properties we had walked through during our whirlwind realty weekend and decided to make an offer on a two-story townhouse in southeast Denver. We were ready to tell our families and our Minnesota friends. They were shocked. For years, they had heard us dream out loud about the possibility of leaving, but none of them ever really thought it would happen. When we put our Minneapolis house on the market, their denial evaporated. And so did their hopes of changing our minds.

Hauling boxes of old kitchen items, vases, games, air conditioners, books, tapes, CDs, and other paraphernalia out of our house for our garage sale stirs within me a curious mixture of longing and purging. People arrived early. How odd it felt to watch strangers walking away with pieces of our lives. Friends stopped by, too, to sit a while and chat, watching buyers come and go, leaving with small mementos of our years together. There is something cleansing about ridding oneself of things that are no longer useful, items that no longer serve a purpose even though once they may have been the most cherished possessions in the household. It's less satisfying to take leave of dear friends, many of whom I'd known for over a decade. It breaks my heart to say good-bye.

I saw my family-practice doctor for a Paxil recheck. I asked her if she thought the added boost of Buspar, a stronger anti-anxiety medication, might ease my clenched throat muscles. "It's worth a try," she agreed. She also suggested that it was time for me to see a specialist. She wanted to ensure that there were no polyps or tumors on my vocal cords causing the speech impairment.

On my doctor's recommendation, I met with an ear-nose-throat (ENT) specialist. The ENT threaded a fiber-optic tube down the back of my throat to get an up-close view of my vocal cords. The procedure was extremely uncomfortable. I gagged as she slid the tube past my uvula. *Can this be necessary?* I asked myself. *This is so barbaric.*

With the tube still inserted down my throat, the ENT asked me to say "e." I gagged. The purpose of this maneuver, she assured me, was to allow her to witness the vibration in my vocal cords as I spoke a variety of vowels, consonants, and short words. The fiber-optic tube also allowed her to see if any polyps or tumors had taken up residence on my vocal cords. Luckily, nothing had homesteaded there.

After the examination, the ENT said that she thought I might have a voice disorder, which she called spasmodic dysphonia. If so, this condition would be causing my vocal cords to tighten when I try to talk. However, ascertaining an exact diagnosis required the skills of an entire team of medical specialists. The ENT referred me to a speech pathologist, then smiled and told me not to worry. "If it is spasmodic dysphonia," she assured, "there is something we can do about it." I didn't even think to ask her what that *something* might be. I took the referral slip and went home, a little sore from the probing examination, but a little hopeful, too.

Might there be a way out of this vocal mess? Didn't that psychic tell me that my voice would return, once I had confronted my mother?

Could this be what she meant?

The next week, I met with a speech pathologist, who conducted a series of non-invasive tests. There wasn't a probing tube in sight, thank god. The speech pathologist asked, "How long have you been experiencing this problem?" And, "What steps have you taken to try to solve it?" I told her about the psychotherapy and the speech therapy. I told her that a speech therapist had diagnosed my problem as tongue placement and had put me through a battery of exercises, all to no avail. She nodded and assured me that spasmodic dysphonia is commonly misdiagnosed. Many medical professionals—including doctors—have never heard of it.

During my session with the speech pathologist, I attempted to read a series of words and sentences. As I struggled through, she listened, analyzing the quality of my speech. She asked me to repeat vowel and consonant sounds. Each time my vocalizations were thwarted by clenching—the same strangled tones I had been experiencing for four years.

At the end of the testing, the speech pathologist told me she thought I had adductor spasmodic dysphonia. Although no one knows what causes this disorder, researchers believe that it involves a region deep in the brain called the basal ganglia. She said that my brain is sending incorrect messages to the muscles controlling the movement of my vocal folds, causing them to contract inappropriately.

191

The speech pathologist told me that, before treatment could begin, I would have to see a neurologist, to ensure that my condition was not neurological. There is no cure, she told me, but there is a way to temporarily relieve the symptoms. She assured me there were others who sounded like me, others who faced the day-to-day struggle of trying to speak with a throttled voice. In a weird way, knowing this made my heart leap! Not that I wished to inflict this hell on anyone else, but now I knew I was not alone. And, best of all, the mystery was solved! My voice problem is *physiologically* based. I have a rare voice disorder. I have spasmodic dysphonia.

I met with the spasmodic dysphonia team at Hennepin County Medical Center in downtown Minneapolis. There I endured another round of invasive testing. First, a different speech pathologist put me through her round of tests. Why, I wondered, didn't she accept the results forwarded to her by the original speech pathologist? Was that not proof enough to satisfy her clinical questions? This second speech pathologist recorded my vocal cord vibrations onto a computer. After she analyzed a printout, she told me she agreed with the first finding—I had spasmodic dysphonia. An extreme case of it, at that.

She sent me off to meet with a neurologist, who conducted his own series of non-invasive tests to rule out neurological damage. Could I raise my left arm? Could I touch the middle finger of my right hand to the tip of my nose? Could I name the President of the United States? Could I say what day of the week it was? Did I feel dizzy? Experience headaches? I must have moved my limbs in just the right way and answered his questions lucidly and factually, because he released me to the next, and final phase, of this three-pronged investigation with a clean bill of neurological health.

Down the busy hospital hall I walked, heading toward the Hennepin County Medical Center's ENT offices. Knowing what lay ahead, I took a deep breath and tried to steady myself. After my original ENT visit, I wasn't looking forward to having a tube threaded down the back of my throat. The diagnostic procedure that awaited me turned out to be even more uncomfortable than the first one had been. This second ENT threaded a fiber-optic tube up my nose then down the back of my throat. I panicked. *Who invented these procedures?* I wanted to yell. *The Marquis de Sade?* And why, again, weren't the findings of the first ENT accepted as proof of my condition?

My fate was sealed. There was no way out of this tube prob-ing, so I tried to breathe and calm myself. As I inhaled and exhaled around the plastic tube, the ENT asked me to sound out vowels and consonants. He handed me a sheet of paper that contained a paragraph of typewritten text and asked me to read it, with the damned tubing still inserted. At last, this second ENT's diagnosis confirmed those of his colleagues. With this official medical stamp of approval, the ENT sent me off to receive my first botox treatment.

The poison becomes the medicine, as Pema Chödrön says. To treat spasmodic dysphonia, the ENT injected a needle through my larynx. It contained a minute, purified quantity of the deadly toxin botulism—which they call botox. He targeted the nearby muscles of the vocal fold. The botox would weaken these, dis-arming their ability to obey the commands sent by my neuro-transmitters to contract. Although the source for this rare voice disorder seems to originate in the brain, treatment is focused at the sight of the contractions. Poison, in the form of botulism bac-terium, becomes the unexpected salve, the solution, the God of Speech, the Returner of Voices.

However, even this warrior is eventually vanquished and the

neurotransmitters reassert their dominance. In time, the botox wears off and the vocal muscle regains its strength, allowing it to respond to the neural signals, and contract again. The amount of the toxin and the length of time between injections varies from person to person. Each patient is assessed and treated, individually. On average, the ENT told me that I could expect to receive injections every three to six months.

The prospect of being stuck in the larynx with a needle filled with toxin did not appeal to me. However, if this was the price I had to pay to get my voice back, I was willing to assent to its rigors. How long I had waited to hear my own clear, sweet voice, to speak without hesitation, to open my mouth and let my words pour forth!

My first injection was daunting. I lay on my back on an examining table in the treatment room with my head tilted over a rounded neck pillow. Images of sacrificial lambs waiting to have their throats slit floated through my mind. I could see the slaughterer's knife poised above the wooly head of the shivering sheep. I could smell the fear. It was mine. I tried to dispel this picture, banish it from my head. It served no purpose other than to increase my already soaring anxiety. I breathed deeply, averting my eyes from the needle that contained my only hope of speech.

Before he administered the botox, the ENT injected lidocaine into my larynx to numb my throat. He also attached a probe to enable him to "see" the vibrations of my vocal muscles. This would help him pinpoint the exact spot in my vocal muscle where the medicine should be injected. He then asked me to make a high "e" vowel sound. The monitor crackled, revealing the spot most in need of the precious botox. The ENT inserted a needle into my larynx. The needle prick stung, in spite of the lidocaine. I felt the cold tip slice through the tight fibers of my vocal folds. Through this slender metal tube, a small amount of botox burrowed its way

194

into the belly of my vocal muscles. It was a beginning. We would have to wait and see how well the medicine took.

After the procedure, I thanked the doctor and shook his hand. Then, I walked five blocks across downtown, to the building where my friend Carol works. I had prearranged for her to drive me home. I had no idea what state I'd be in after the botox, but remembering how I had felt after the original testing procedure at the initial ENT's office the month before, I decided to err on the side of comfort. I waited in the lobby of my friend's work place. As Carol descended the staircase to the main floor, I burst into tears and ran to her. She hugged me. All the fear and anxiety I had swallowed during the botox procedure flooded through me, released at last. I felt violated. Old incest wounds howled. I felt small, fearful, and out of control.

After all these years of not knowing, I finally have a name and a reason for my strangled voice. I have reluctantly joined the ranks of the approximately 50,000 people in North America—sixty percent of whom are women—who have this rare voice disorder known as spasmodic dysphonia.

The Hennepin County ENT had told me what to expect. The day after a botox injection I would begin to experience a breathy voice. This was an indication that the medicine had taken effect. The result was an airy, Marilyn Monroe sounding voice—something I would later describe as Melanie Griffith imitating Minnie Mouse. This breathiness would last from one to two weeks. Eventually it would give way to my normal voice, until the botox wore off. Then the vocal tightening would return. At that point, another injection would be scheduled.

My first injection proved to have a less than desirable outcome. I was breathy for a few days, but not excessively so. To my grave disappointment, my voice never returned to normal. When

I called my ENT to report in, he suggested that perhaps he hadn't given me a large enough dose. At his prompting, I scheduled a booster shot. I had questioned whether or not I should start treatments in Minnesota when I was planning to move to Denver in less than a month, but the Hennepin County ENT thought it best to begin because my condition was so severe. He wanted to try to provide me with some vocal relief before I moved and found a new ENT to take over my care. He assured me that the first year of treatment was a process of trial and error. We could begin, but my Denver doctor would work with me to find the correct dose, with the least amount of side effects, for my particular condition. I prayed that the impending booster shot would hold me over until I could get help in Denver. That first injection was a lot of physical discomfort for such little gain.

Two days after my botox booster shot, I felt relieved. The second treatment worked much better than the initial dose. Within a day, I experienced a slight breathiness, though nothing excessive. By the second day, it was also easier to talk, although my speech had yet to return to what I remember, as normal. Maybe, in time, a dosage can be found that will change all that. I prayed that the ENTs in Denver would be as adept as those in Minneapolis.

Jane and I had dinner with my mom and my stepfather. Our dinner together was a going-away event, one of many that Jane and I had scheduled before our departure on August 4th. Surprisingly I felt strong about seeing Mom. Dining in public in a nice restaurant felt like neutral ground. I hadn't seen my mother since our March therapy session, four months before. I had spoken with her on the phone a few times since our meeting, even though I had stressed that I wanted to communicate solely through e-mail. But I decided telling her about my move to

Colorado was best done on the phone, not in cyberspace. I had made the rule; I could bend it when I thought it made sense to do so.

Over pasta and salad, Jane and I told my mother and stepfather about our new townhouse in Denver. I also told them about my voice disorder and the botox treatments. They both commented that my voice sounded better than it had in years. They were happy that I had discovered the reason for my troubles and a way to manage the condition.

To my surprise, our dinner conversation was easy. Mom displayed no apparent resentment about having been put through the rigors of our therapy session. To my delight, she acted like a responsible grown-up. And so did I. I didn't spiral into old memories of mistrust. I held fast to my newfound adult sensibility. The vulnerable six-year-old who usually accompanied me on such outings was nowhere to be found. I'd left her, secure, in the imaginary arms of a loving and attentive caregiver, so she wouldn't have to doubt the love in her mother's eyes as she sat across the restaurant table, saying good-bye to her.

Before we left to go home in our separate cars, my mother asked if she could visit Jane and me in Denver. I told her I would let her know when I was ready. My words were refreshingly direct and totally devoid of meanness. Without blame or shame, I simply stated how I felt and in doing so, I found no need to harbor anger or grief.

In collecting estimates from moving van companies, I learned that things are charged by estimated weight. A guy comes to the house, looks at your furniture, the number of rooms to pack, then estimates the total weight of all your household goods. The moving fee is computed from these calculations. It's strange how one's entire life can be synthesized into 6,000 pounds, $2,500. Years of making love, fighting, making up, laughing, dancing, tears, and joy, and furniture rearranging—distilled into a dollar amount. Does life get more concrete than that?

Jane and I hosted a "Moving to Denver" open house. We invited friends, neighbors, co-workers, and family members. The day was long, physically exhausting, and emotionally draining. Hugs were abundant. Tears were, too. It was hard to witness people's sadness over our leaving. It was poignant as well. We touched and were touched by many loving women and men. Jane had lived in Minnesota for over twenty years. It had been my home for nearly thirty, but something calls me to Denver. I'm not sure what, exactly; I know only that it feels like the next step of a very long and serpentine path.

At our going-away party, friends commented on my voice. Some, who hadn't known about the recent diagnosis, asked if I had a cold. Ugly, old shame surged. My face reddened, and I muttered, "No," but provided no further explanation. I couldn't find the courage. Too many emotions were careening through my heart that day to ferret out the reasons for my still-clenching voice. How could I tell them that the botox wasn't working as well as I wanted? I could hardly bear the truth of it. The magic poison wasn't potent enough. Would this always be so? Or could I trust that finding the correct dose was a process, as surely as any of the other processes I had struggled through all these long four years. It would take a while, the ENT told me, until the right combination of botox seeped into my vocal muscles and silenced the contractions, but I felt so impatient, so near to a solution and yet so far from a workable resolution.

I tried to remind myself to have compassion as I adjusted to the medication and to the fact that I'd finally found a reason for my speech problems. I told myself to believe in the possibility of a normal voice. The doctors and the speech pathologists had no reason to lie, no reason to feed me false hope. Time is what I needed. Time and patience. Then the huge boulder of doubt would be lifted from my heart.

When moving day arrived, I could hardly contain my joy. The day of all days had finally come. I was leaving Minnesota.

The van arrived early in the morning, and the movers loaded up by late afternoon. They would meet us in Colorado in four days. By early evening, Jane and I crawled into my blue Mazda, and headed south on I-35 on our way to our new home. After two days on the road, we shrieked with glee as the first glimpse of mountain peaks emerged from the blur of prairie and sky. We sped along the long stretch of I-76 westbound and arrived in Denver hours later, waving to the outline of Pikes Peak to the south, Mount Evans to the west. We maneuvered through thick city traffic, and turned, finally, into the driveway of our Denver townhouse. Tired from the road and craving a hot bath and some good food, Jane and I opened the door to our new home and stepped inside. Our road-weary eyes were stunned by the absence of the rich, oak woodwork that we had left behind in our Minneapolis house. Instead, empty rooms, aching for furniture, greeted us. Naked wooden floors cried for throw rugs. Blank walls begged for artwork. And a god-awful, textured ceiling stared down on our astonished heads. Certain that our move had been a mistake, we promptly left and drove to our friends' house for comfort. Their coaching helped. It would take time, they reminded us. And we would feel better after the moving van arrived, and we could fill the spaces with our own stuff.

Our friends loaned us the futon from their couch so we could sleep on the floor in our new living room until our furniture arrived. That night, as we looked up at the speckled ceiling, I was reminded of the apartment building in North St. Paul into which my mother, stepfather, sisters, and I had moved in 1967. Back then, I thought such ceilings were the height of style—a symbol that we had made it. Their textured surfaces were a far cry from the cracked plaster walls and ceilings of the sagging old house we had left behind in my hometown in western New York. Now in Denver, those textured ceilings sent me reeling into a retro time warp I wasn't quite sure I appreciated.

Our friends had been right. We felt immeasurably better after our furniture arrived. Next came the challenge of living amid stacks of sealed boxes. As we opened cartons and unwrapped dishes and other items, we found that our Minneapolis friends had written on crate-wrapping paper. "Hello Jane and Mary. We miss you." We were thrilled by their thoughtfulness—the surprise notes from loved ones amidst the boxed contents of our lives.

Soon after our arrival, Jane had to return to Minneapolis for three weeks to tie up loose ends at her old office. Hanging pictures would have to wait until she came back. In spite of the presence of dressers and chairs, the house felt emptier without her, but the couch, nestled in front of the stone fireplace, assured me she'd be back. The Amish oak table stood solidly in our new dining room, filling me with a sense of place and purpose. Its familiar surface would cradle our plates and silverware here as well as in Minneapolis. Little by little, the Denver house was beginning to feel like home.

Two weeks after Jane had returned to Minneapolis, I flew back to meet her and help her drive our Honda to Denver. During my brief stay in the Twin Cities, I visited the ENT at Hennepin County Medical Center to receive another botox treatment. It had been almost six weeks since my initial shot. I kept my hopes high that this time the injection would produce quantifiable results. I wanted my voice back, and I wasn't happy that this supposed miracle drug was failing to deliver on its promise. I hated not knowing how long it would take before the medicine would kick in and I would be able to speak without strain. Impatience hovered like a hungry buzzard.

It would be ridiculous to travel between Denver and Minneapolis every time I needed a botox injection, so my Minnesota doctor referred me to a colleague in Denver. On a bright October morning, I met with Dr. Karen Rhew. She conducted a voice evaluation and once more I endured the fiber-optic scope threaded up my nose and down my throat. However, this time Dr. Rhew showed me my vocal cords in the video monitor. I was struck by how similar they looked to a vaginal opening, soft and pink, fleshy and wet. They contracted and expanded as I tried to speak with the probe down my throat. In an amazing quirk of nature, the human body's sacred parts—the vocal cords, the vagina—resembled each other. Was there a connection between the silencing of sexual abuse and the silencing of spasmodic dysphonia?

Before she became a physician, Dr. Rhew earned a master's degree in speech pathology. During a stint at the National Institute of Health, she contributed five years of research on spasmodic dysphonia. I was relieved to learn that she also had very definite, holistic ideas on how to treat this rare disorder. She strongly advocated voice therapy as a way to teach her patients how to re-train their voices and use proper breathing techniques. She believed that this alleviated the stress placed upon the vocal cords and prolonged the effects of the botox injection. She also prescribed a regimen of vitamins to provide my muscles and my nervous system with internal support.

In November of 1997 I had my first botox shot with Dr. Rhew. While the Minnesota ENTs injected the medication into the muscles on each side of the larynx, Dr. Rhew preferred to inject only one side at a time—left or right. Alternate sides were treated each visit. This approach is less harsh to the vocal muscles over time and results in fewer side effects, such as increased trouble swallowing. Dr. Rhew had upped my dose, injecting the vocal muscles on the left side of my throat with 6.0 units of botox. One week post-treatment, my voice was unmistakably breathy. That was the sign I had waited for. I knew that the longer I was breathy, the longer I would experience the long-hoped-for return of my normal voice.

This time the shot took.

On December 5th, 1997, my voice was NORMAL!!! For the first time in over four years, I could speak without strain or struggle, without grasping or clenching. My voice was clear and loud and strong. Hallelujah!

Ironically, words can not adequately describe my elation. The strangled sound was stilled; the tense speech was softened. The strained muscles were eased. I felt whole again. A full-voiced member of the human race. Oh, what joy! What boundless happiness! And gratitude. Deep and abiding gratitude!

Epilogue

The ENT at the Hennepin County Medical Center told me that spasmodic dysphonia (SD) is not psychogenic. He said that oftentimes this disorder is misdiagnosed or not diagnosed immediately because it is mistakenly thought that the voice dysfunction has psychological roots. He said that there is no evidence that SD patients have experienced psychological trauma any more so than what presents in the wider culture. However, researchers aren't fully certain of what does cause the neurotransmitters in the basal ganglia to run amok.

I am not a medical researcher, but I do not entirely agree with the doctors and the scientists who claim that SD is merely a physiological, medical condition. When I look back on my life and how silenced I was to my own self-worth and my own truth, this voice disorder makes a certain kind of sense. It is no mere fluke that an emotional/spiritual trauma would manifest itself in a physical, bodily way—affecting the weakest link in my physiological chain.

For me, that weak link happened to be the neurotransmitters in my basal ganglia that control the motor movement of my vocal muscles.

That this physical manifestation was triggered as I wrote my first novel was also no mere coincidence. Writing *No Matter What* rattled the parts of my body that weren't ready to go public. My cellular memory knew only how to constrict, shut down, be silent. I was born prematurely, before my nervous system finished its maturation process. As an infant and as a child, I was exposed to external stimuli that I had difficulty processing—my parents' arguing, the loudness of fighting, the emotional undertow of my parents' grief, my brothers' anger, the sexual abuse. As an intuitive kid, I had a difficult time processing the internal effects of this external commotion. I learned how to contract when I sensed danger or harm. It doesn't surprise me that a part of my nervous system was affected. Years later, when it was safe enough to let go, my body responded in the only way it knew—by contracting.

My voice was the ground-zero site. For someone else the body-mind-spirit might have responded through cancer or MS or fibromyalgia. It matters little how body memories manifest. What became increasingly clear to me is that they do. Body/mind/spirit are a unified organism. What touches one touches all.

After fitful tries, my botox dosage is finally regulated. At long last my healing journey has come to a place of stillness and resolution. The long years of intensive psychotherapy and bodywork—

along with my clay sculptures, drawings, and dreamwork—had transported me to the other side. In facing my personal demons, in learning to befriend my fear and my anger, my grief and my sorrow, I was able to reclaim the wholeness of my life, in ways that I had never before dreamed possible.

Was it difficult? Extremely so. Was it worth the effort? Undeniably. The path I chose led me back to my truest Self—not a perfect person devoid of quirks and neuroses, but, instead, a perfectly flawed woman with goodness and selfishness co-existing in her imperfectly human heart.

What I gained most from my journey was a surer sense of my voice. The irony of losing the ability to speak without strain is that I uncovered a multitude of voices I had not before recognized. As I struggled to speak, I learned to shout out my deepest names—writer, artist, lover, friend, warrior, healer, incest survivor. I discovered strength and courage when I was most vulnerable and fearful. I learned that I am a soft-bellied warrior, brave and resilient. It is never too late to call oneself home, to clean up one's messy heart, to open oneself to the love and compassion of others. To risk everything is to gain a richness of love, a tenderness of witness that nothing in my life had prepared me for.

Voice is a particular gift—a singular identity, rather like the DNA of one's soul. I learned that there are many ways to speak, many voices in each human being. What is most essential is to claim yours—and share it with others. What this world needs most is for each of us to give voice to our lives, to break the silence of lies and half-truths. To stand in the fullness of who we deeply are and speak, without hesitation, in a voice loud and insistent.

Doors open when one dares to risk the un-riskable. In March of 1998, I received a letter from a woman named Edvige Giunta, who had read *No Matter What*. Edvige, I would soon learn, was a literature professor, a scholar and a writer who teaches at Jersey City University in Jersey City, New Jersey. She had happened upon my novel after requesting a literary search of titles by Italian American women. Edvige wrote to tell me that she loved *No Matter What* and wished to talk with me about the book in the hopes of including me in her ongoing scholarship on contemporary Italian American women writers.

I replied to Edvige's letter and soon we were talking on the phone. At that time, she graciously asked me to submit a proposal to participate on a panel at the American Italian Historical Association (AIHA) annual conference, which was scheduled for November 1998 in New York City. The theme of the conference was politics and ethnicity. I told her I would submit one of my memoir pieces from my manuscript-in-progress, *A Talk with the Moon.*

My proposal was accepted, and so I found myself traveling to New York City in the fall of 1998 to participate on a panel entitled "Memory Politics." The day before I was scheduled to arrive at La Guardia, Edvige called. She asked me to stand in for a writer who was not able to fulfill her commitment to participate in a literary reading on the final night of the conference.

Much to my amazement, I spontaneously responded, "Yes!"

This would be my first venture into public speaking since I had lost—and found—my voice. I worked closely with Dr. Rhew, my otolaryngologist, to insure that my botox treatment schedule would afford me a strong, clear voice for my conference appearances. Now that my speaking voice would not be a recognizable concern, I would be able to test my emotional resiliency, as well.

I arrived in New York City a few days before the conference, to orient myself to the city and to explore the Big Apple—a place to which I had never before been. I wandered around the city, walking up and down Mid-Town for hours—seeing all the usual tourist sights. To my great discouragement, my beautiful, perfect, clear voice did not take kindly to my excursions. I developed a congestion, which settled into my throat. And while I did not experience the strained, strangled speech that is characteristic of spasmodic dysphonia, I was not to enjoy the strong voice for which I had prepared so diligently.

The first day of the conference, my congestion was quite evident. I consumed massive quantities of herbal tea, throat lozenges, and vegetables, hoping to boost my immune system and circumvent a cold. I left the evening reception early to return to my hotel room to rest and restore for the following day. I told myself that I would not let this voice congestion interfere. I refused to allow this setback to come between me and my first public reading in four years. Being at this conference, meeting these amazing Italian American women writers, scholars, poets, artists, and filmmakers was too important an experience to not give it my best.

Back in my hotel room, I called Jane and sobbed. I felt disappointed and angry that my voice wasn't perfect, as planned. I knew I was not going to let the inadequacy of congestion ruin my re-emergence. However, I felt cheated by fate, angry at my voice disorder. By the end of our conversation, I felt resolved to go forward, do my readings, inform my audiences that I had caught a cold, and not give up on myself. My voice wasn't perfect, but maybe it didn't need to be. Maybe this was another huge lesson, in a long string of lessons that brought me closer to the realization that I couldn't control things, even though I desperately wanted to. This conference was the opportunity I had waited for—the chance to read my work to an audience who understood its cultural underpinnings.

The next morning, I bought an extra-large cup of chamomile tea and went to the conference armed with more throat lozenges.

207

My first reading—the panel on "Memory Politics"—was shaky. I pre-warned my audience of my vocal congestion and plodded through, taking sips of water when my throat became parched. At one point, one of the audience members, a newfound friend, suggested that I speak into the microphone so as not to strain unnecessarily. I took his advice and completed my reading. I had cleared the first hurdle. It hadn't been a perfect reading, from a voice standpoint, but I had managed to stand before an audience and read my work. And that was an immeasurable victory to me.

Later that evening, on the way to the literary reading, I silently re-affirmed my decision to dig deep and give the best performance I was capable of at the time, in spite of my vocal distress.

Edvige introduced me, and I stood before the crowded room. I took a deep breath, and I explained to the audience that a bit of New York had settled into my throat. I asked them to bear with me. I stuffed a throat lozenge into my cheek and began. The sentences flowed out of me. I connected with the energy of *No Matter What* and gave a fine reading. I felt confident. Giddy with success. My voice, while a bit hoarse, was strong and powerful. *I had done it.* I had faced the fear, hurdled the challenge, and reclaimed my right to read my work in public—with *any* voice that showed up.

When at last I read the final sentence, I closed my book and thanked the audience for listening. I let their applause settle into my bones, and I smiled. I had come full circle. My voice had *not* been silenced. I had survived the years of not knowing, of doubt and fear. After four long years, my writing voice and my speaking voice had been reunited. I settled back into my chair, and listened to the marvelous voices of the other writers as they read their work.

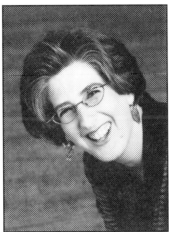

Mary Saracino lives in Denver, Colorado. Her first novel, *No Matter What*, was a 1994 Minnesota Book Award Fiction finalist. Her second novel, *Finding Grace* won the Colorado Authors' League 1999 "Top Hand" Award in the Adult Fiction, Mainsteam/ Literary category. Her memoir/essay, "Valentino, Puglia and Seneca Falls" earned the 2000 Salvator & Margaret Bonomo Prize for Literature. Her work has appeared in numerous literary and cultural journals.